MASTER MANDALAS
Stained Glass Inspiration
by REN

Part of the Ren Collection • **RenCollection.org** • © 2016 All rights reserved by the author/artist
ISBN 978-1-5238-8689-0

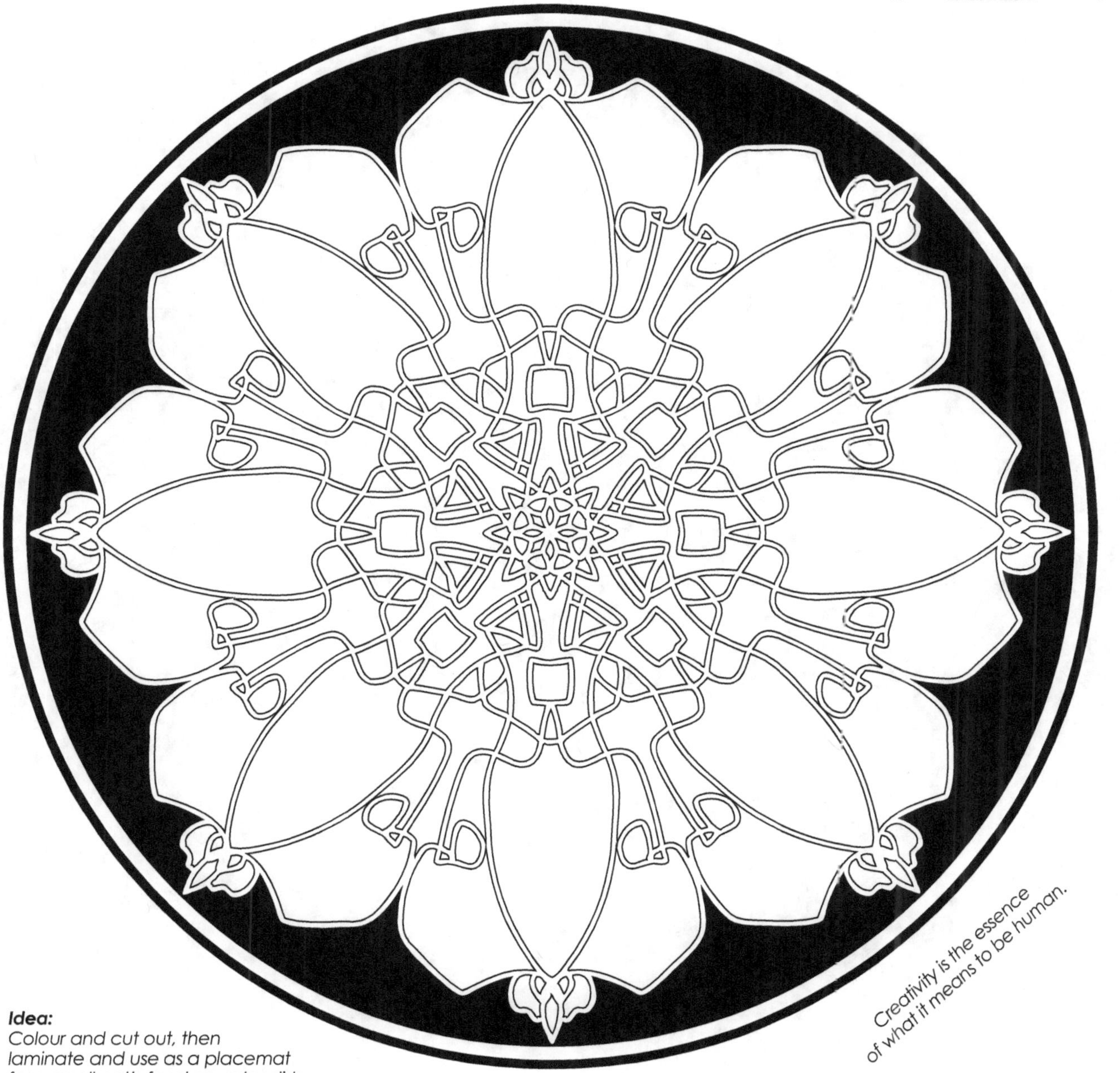

Idea:
Colour and cut out, then
laminate and use as a placemat
for a small pet's food or water dish

*Creativity is the essence
of what it means to be human.*

MASTER MANDALAS
Stained Glass Inspiration by REN

Idea:
Colour and cut out this design; insert a photo or drawing in the centre; laminate for durability

There is no wrong way to colour.

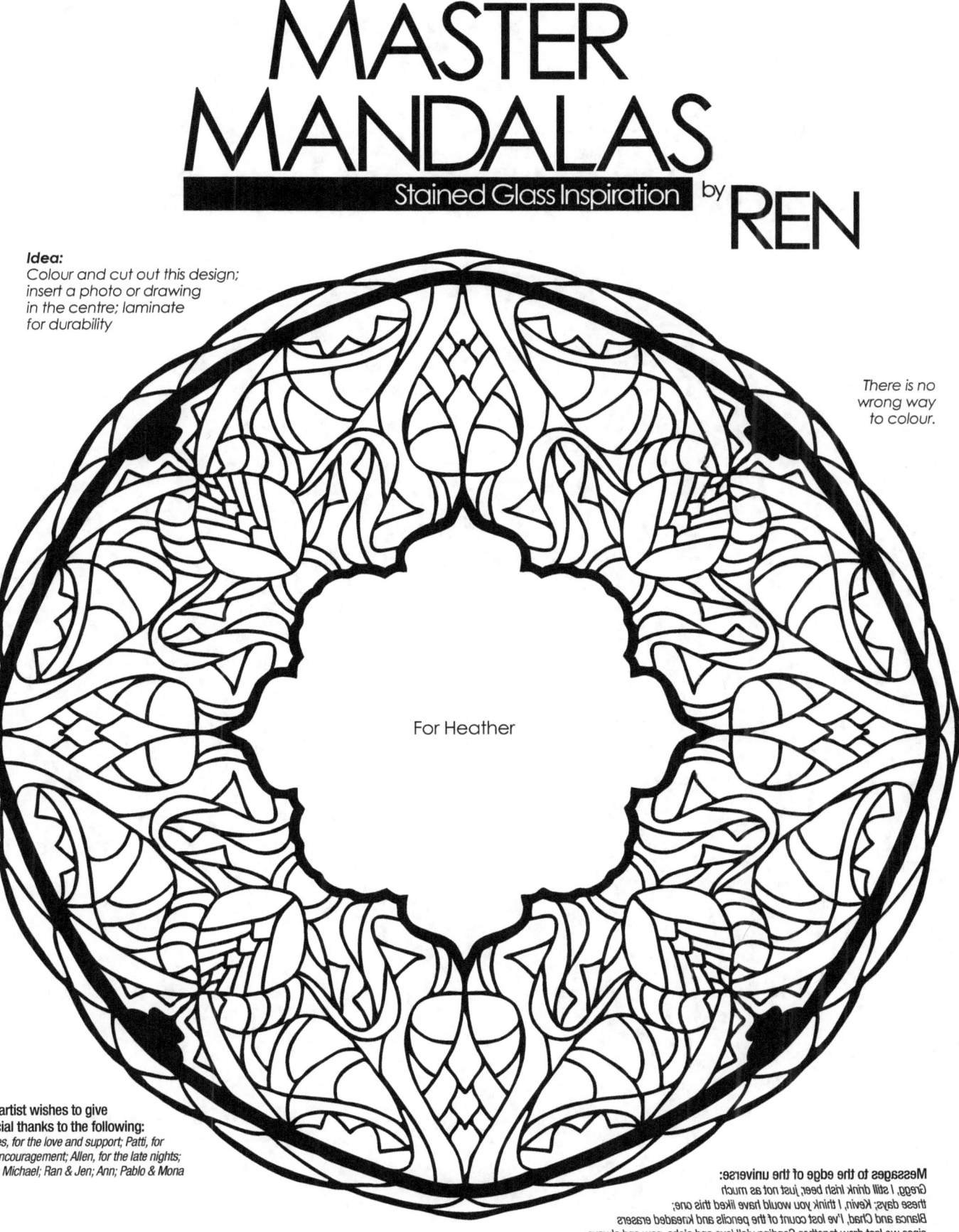

For Heather

The artist wishes to give special thanks to the following:
James, for the love and support; Patti, for the encouragement; Allen, for the late nights; Jess; Michael; Ran & Jen; Ann; Pablo & Mona

Messages to the edge of the universe:
Gregg, I still drink Irish beer, just not as much these days; Kevin, I think you would have liked this one; Blanca and Chad, I've lost count of the pencils and kneaded erasers since we last drew together. Sending y'all love and aloha, now and always.
—R

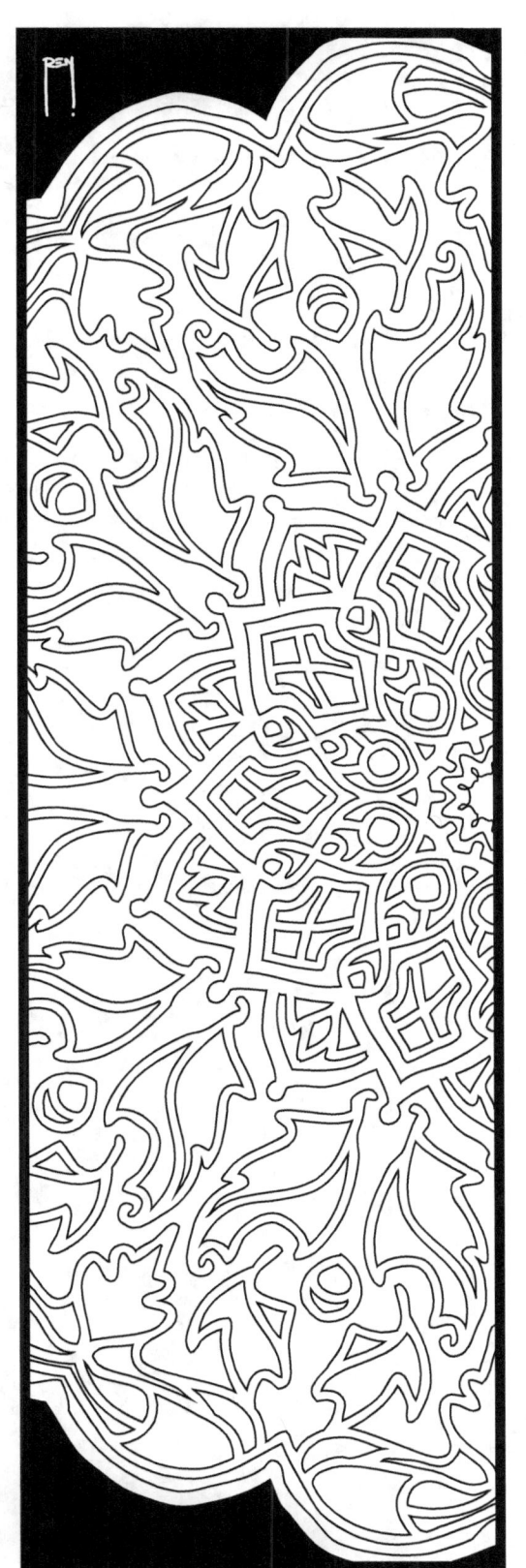

INTRODUCTION

Making of a Master

It's not the mandalas that are the master, it's you: the reader; the colourist; the artist; the creative. Encoded within your DNA is the desire to express your thoughts and feelings, to make a mark in this world.

Too many people say they're not creative, when, in fact, creativity is the essence of what it means to be human. Own it. Explore the world of colour by making marks within these pages. If you make a mistake, then see it as a happy accident, and keep playing with colour.

What to Expect

If you're familiar with mandalas, then you'll know to expect art that fits within a circular (or close to it) shape. In addition, there are lots of bookmarks for you to colour and cut out, maybe even laminate for durability; and there are even more medallions, which make great portable colouring projects; and when they're finished they can be used in various ways, such as scrapbooking, rubber stamping, and/or collage. This book also contains lots of heavy line work, reminiscent of stained glass piping, which makes it easier to keep colours within the boundaries.

More than Lines

This book is about more than just colouring in the lines. It also has encouraging affirmations, thoughts for reflection, and ideas for your finished creations.

I've included these in the book for a number of reasons; the most important is because there was a time when I could have used a resource just like this. A while back, an auto accident left me with a brain injury and memory loss; I was unable to create any visual art for nearly three years — as a creative professional, this was devastating. I would have benefitted greatly from being exposed to abstract images such as these; from practising fine motor skills, such as colouring, in a safe environment; and having positive and encouraging words in my peripheral vision, even if I wasn't able to read them and remember what I had just read. It would have helped me to feel better, if only for a moment.

Everything in this book is here to help you, or someone you love, heal. Even if you don't have any physical injuries or limitations, sometimes our spirit is hurt and needs some time and space to heal as well.

Live bravely, and give back often,
– Ren

Has this book helped you? I'd love to hear from you.
Write to me at RenCollection@gmx.com.

THE CONCEPT OF EVERYTHING

The Insatiable Want for It All

A lifetime ago, I worked in the world of advertising. People like me would sit in sleek meeting rooms, deciding for the consumer what was "beautiful" or "in," and, more importantly, we'd sell things that you *have to have*, right now, more than anything in the world.

It's strange, now, to reflect upon that time, to know and understand the human need to collect — to hoard — absolutely everything. We want a flat stomach, a fat wallet, children who are gifted at being gifted, tons of followers on all the social networks for us to ignore. We want good hair and artisanal food. We want perfect microwave omelettes.

We want everything.

But "everything" is just a concept, and we can never have *everything*, nor should we want it. It's too much. What we can do, however, is to think about what are the few, truly important things in our lives, and focus on that.

We can be grateful for what we already have, for the people who treat us with love and respect, and for the good fortune that art and creativity can provide. What else are *you* grateful for?

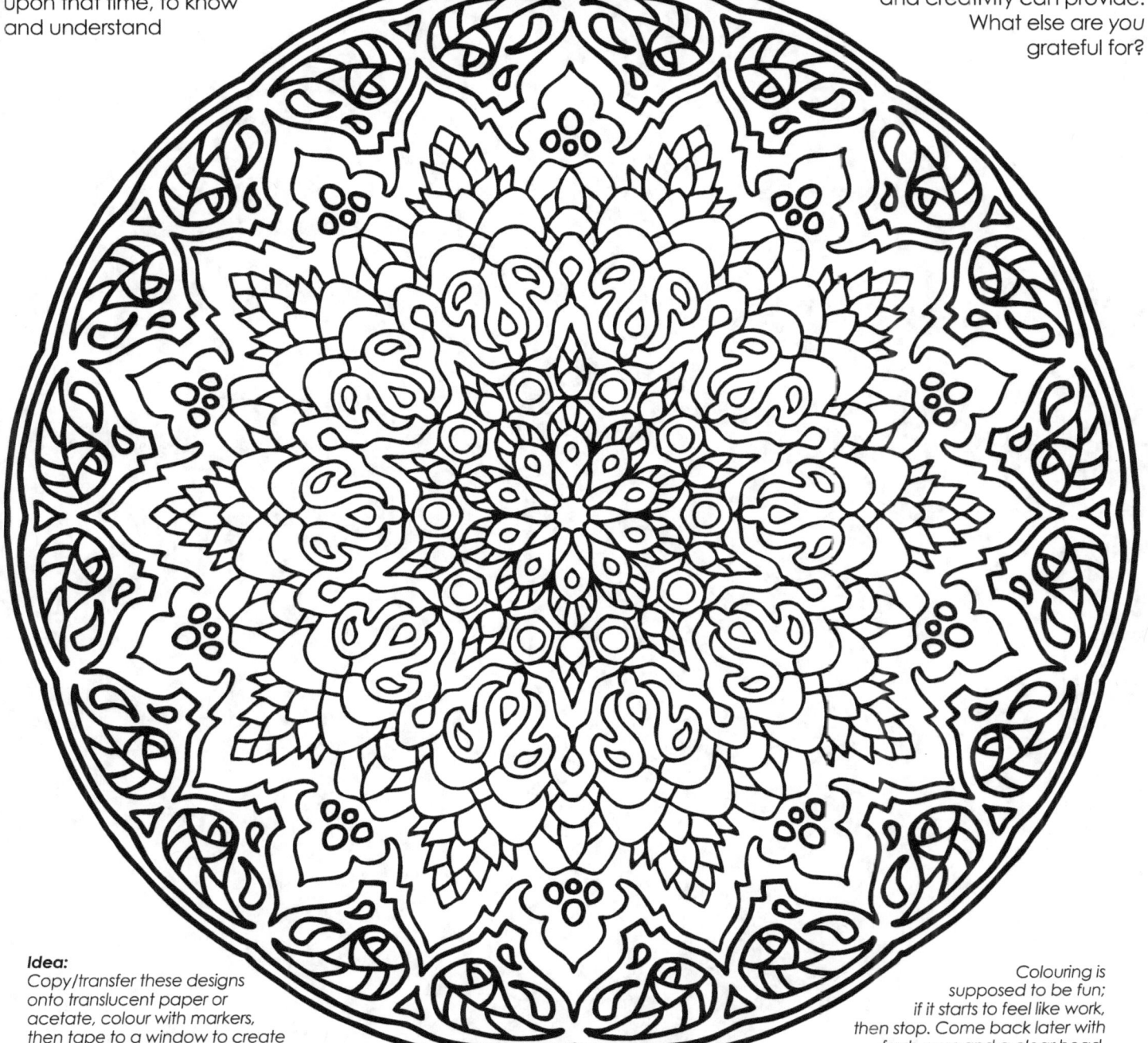

Idea:
Copy/transfer these designs onto translucent paper or acetate, colour with markers, then tape to a window to create stunning faux stained glass

Colouring is supposed to be fun; if it starts to feel like work, then stop. Come back later with fresh eyes and a clear head.

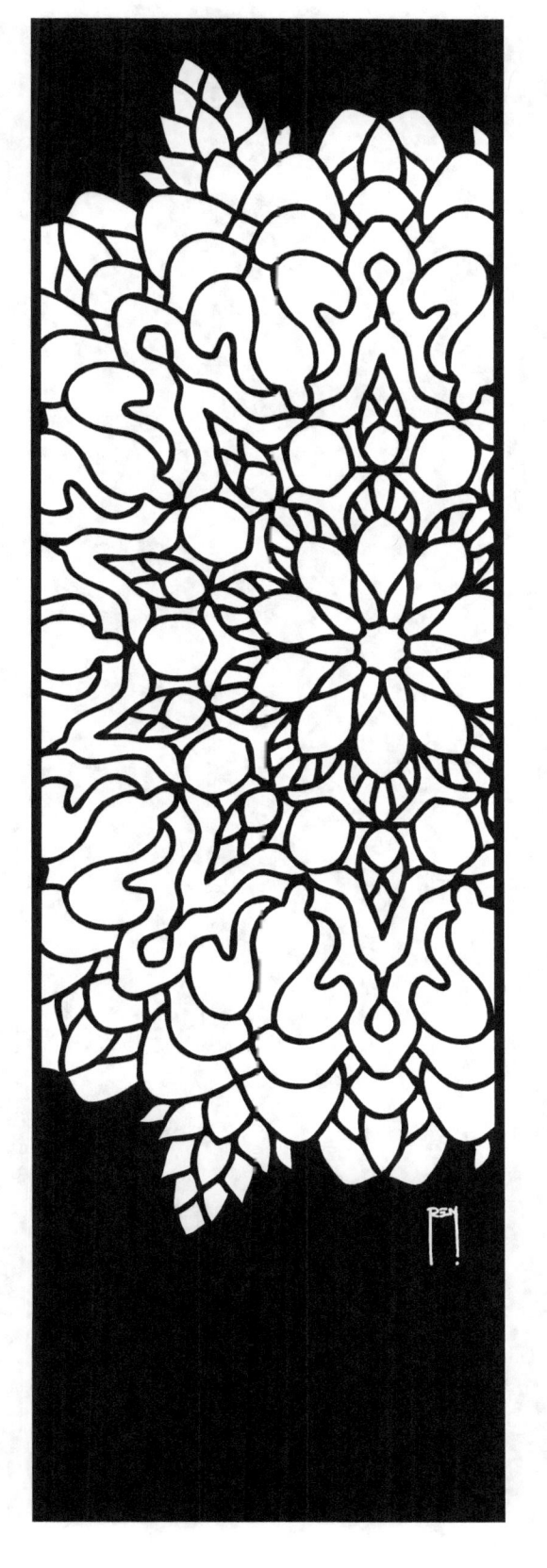
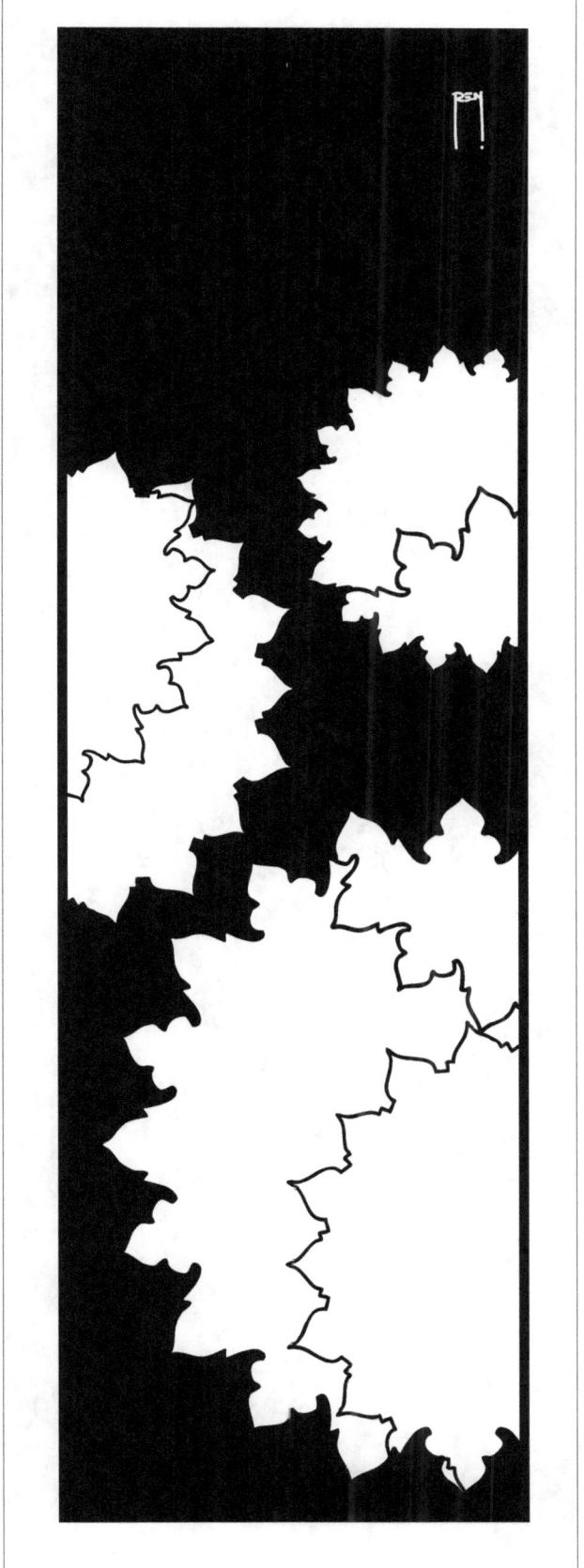

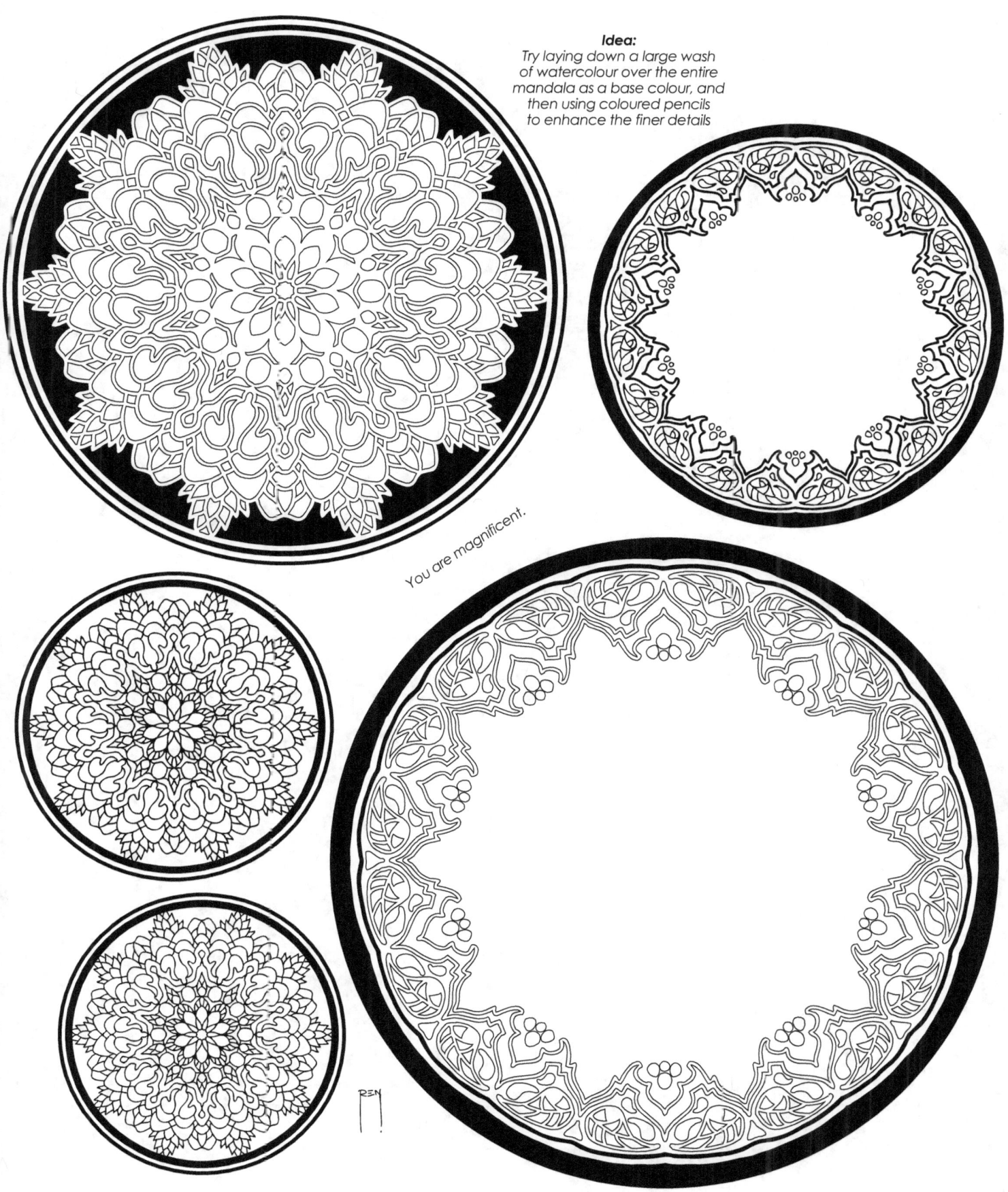

Idea:
Try laying down a large wash of watercolour over the entire mandala as a base colour, and then using coloured pencils to enhance the finer details

You are magnificent.

THE WONDERS OF TIME

The Power of the Intangible

After my brain injury, I swore I had developed the ability to see time: it moved in swirls around every person, animal, plant, and anything else that could wither or decay. People looked like blossoming flowers, showing every possible past, present, and future simultaneously; and with every move they made, the flowers would change shape, size, and intensity.

While in this fractured state, I saw that time could be manipulated, sped up, or slowed down. Different organisms exist at different rates — there really *are* dog years! Dog flowers are bluer than people flowers, which are more lavender; iron skillets are yellow; fabrics are red.

As my brain healed, the blossoming flowers gradually faded and then eventually disappeared. People weren't lavender anymore; dogs weren't blue or cerulean. Things were grey and tepid; the electricity had gone out.

I never thought much about time before I was injured; only when I was able to glimpse its mesmerising colours did I understand humankind's fascination with the concept.

What would you imagine are the colours in your time flower? When would you want to speed up or slow time?

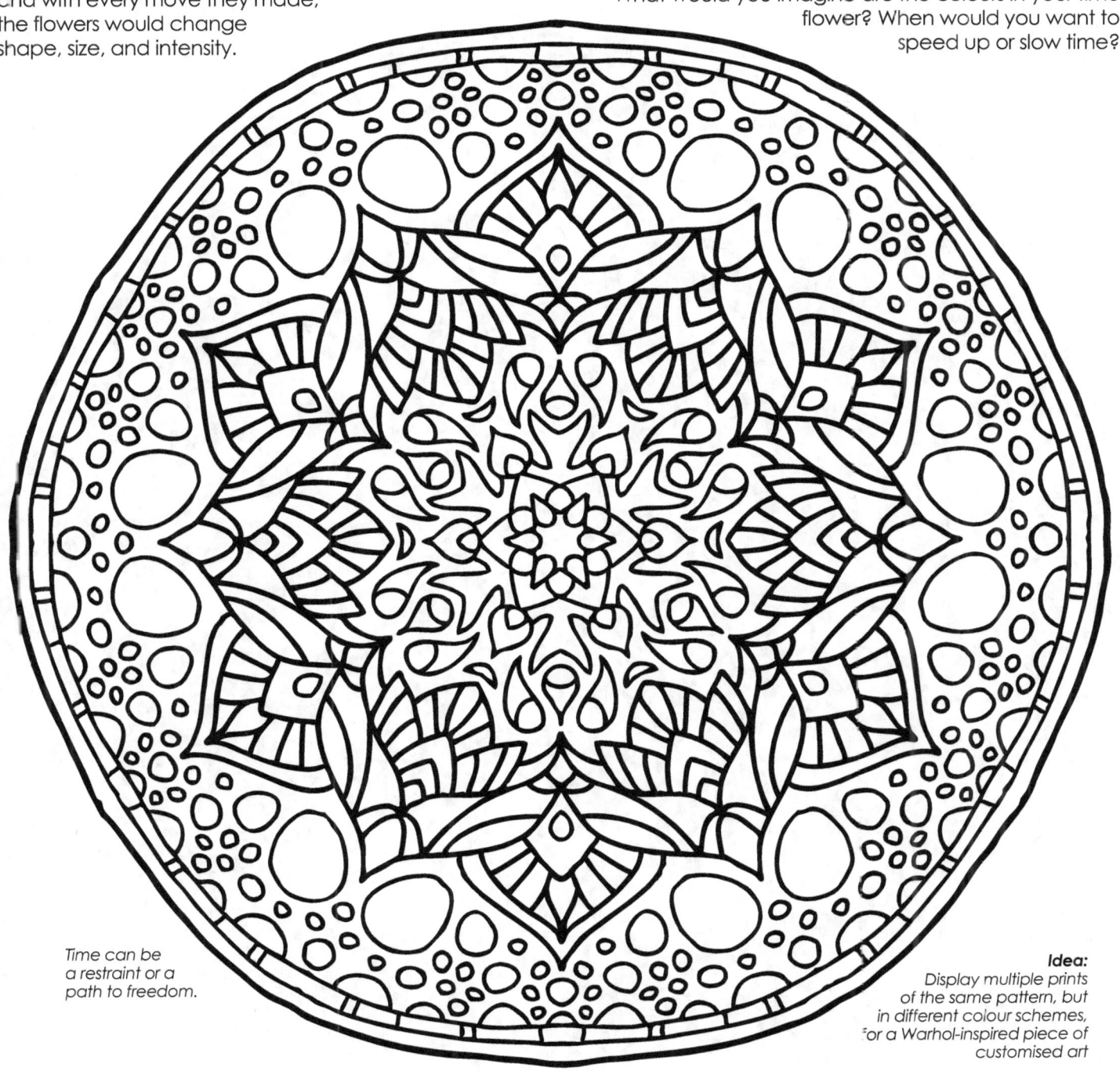

Time can be a restraint or a path to freedom.

Idea:
Display multiple prints of the same pattern, but in different colour schemes, for a Warhol-inspired piece of customised art

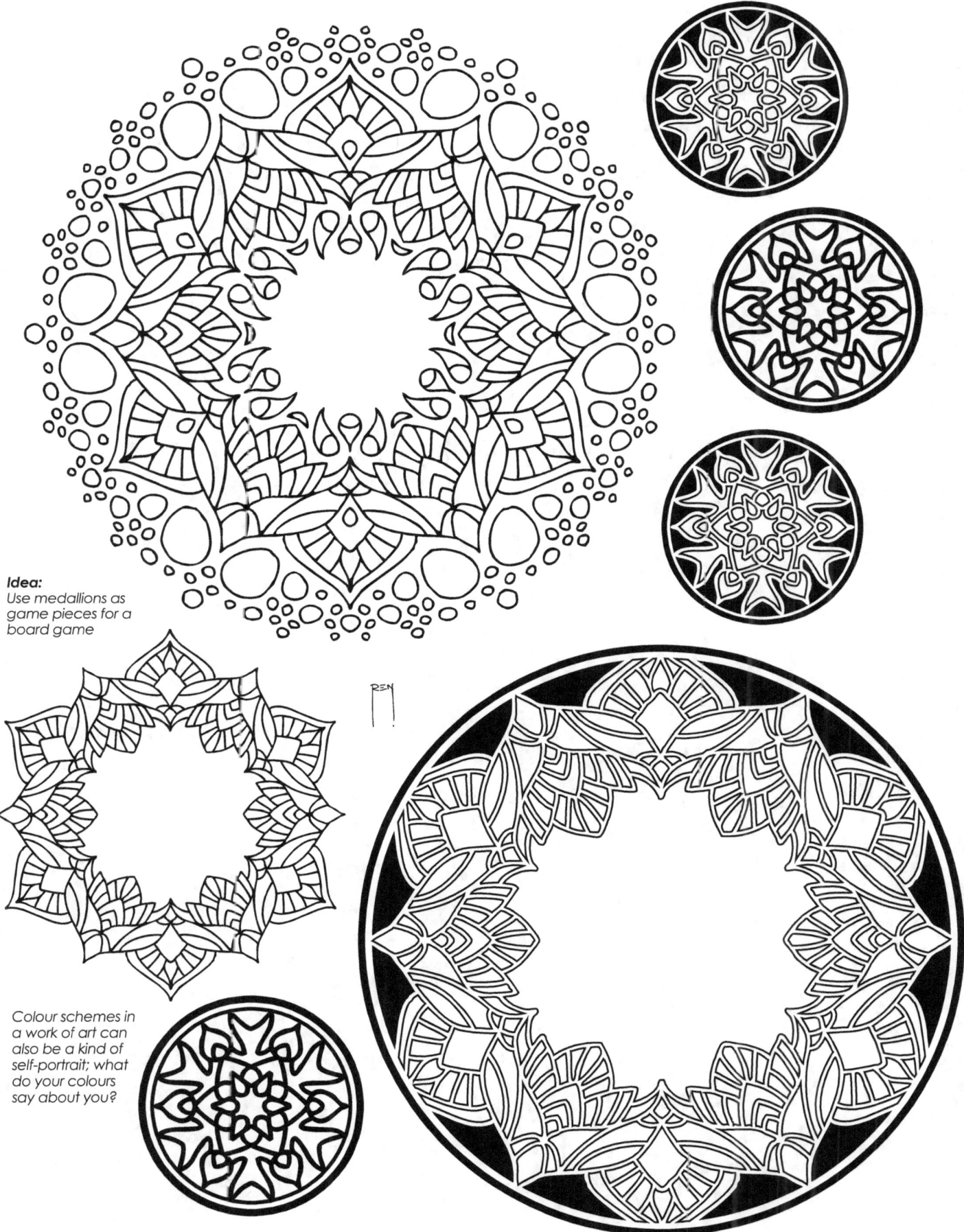

Idea:
Use medallions as game pieces for a board game

Colour schemes in a work of art can also be a kind of self-portrait; what do your colours say about you?

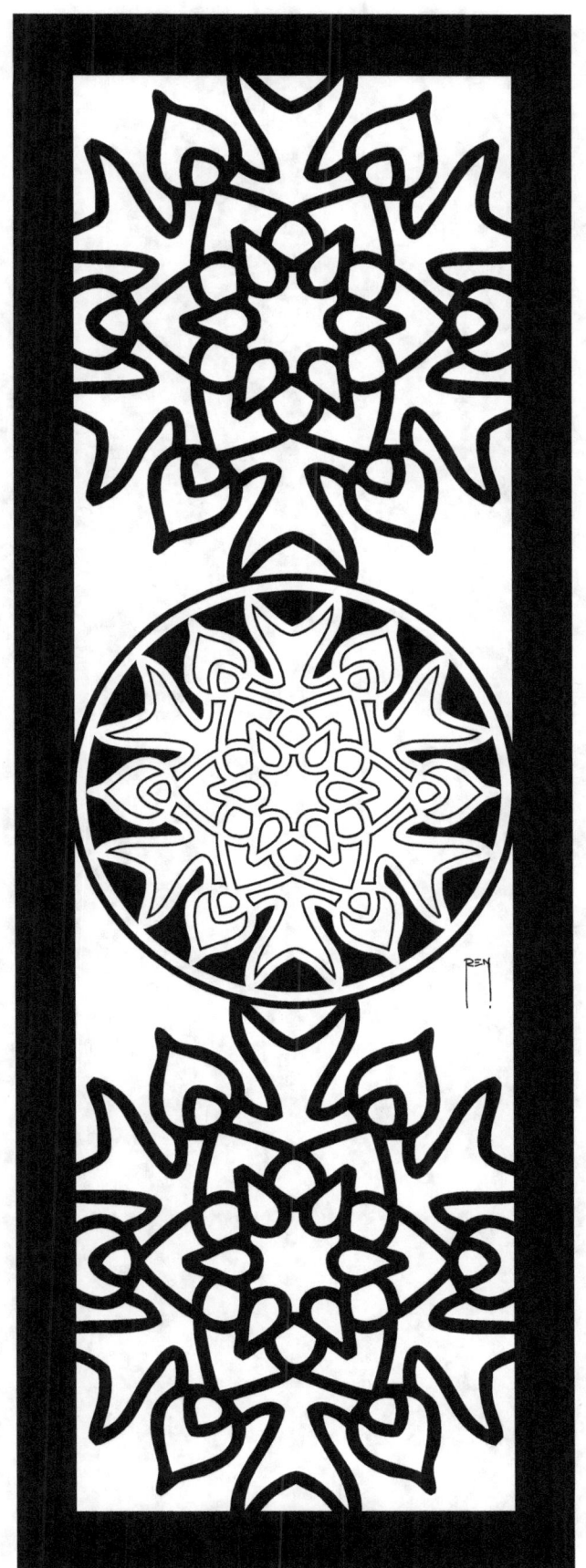
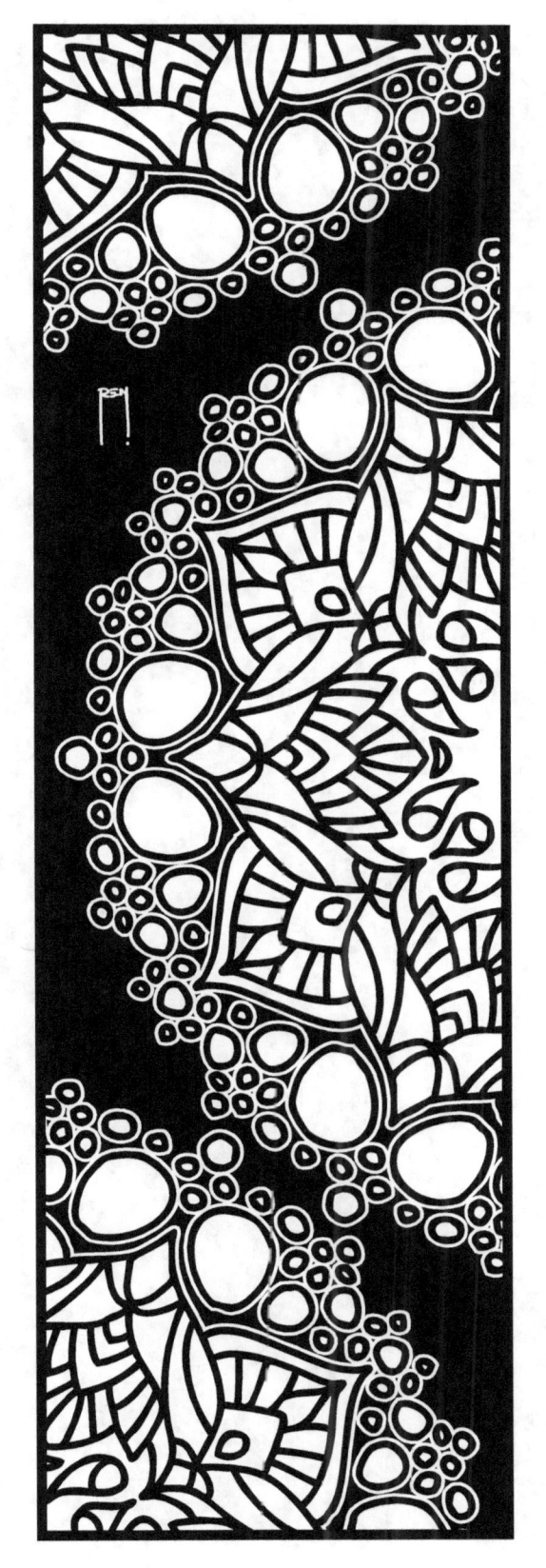

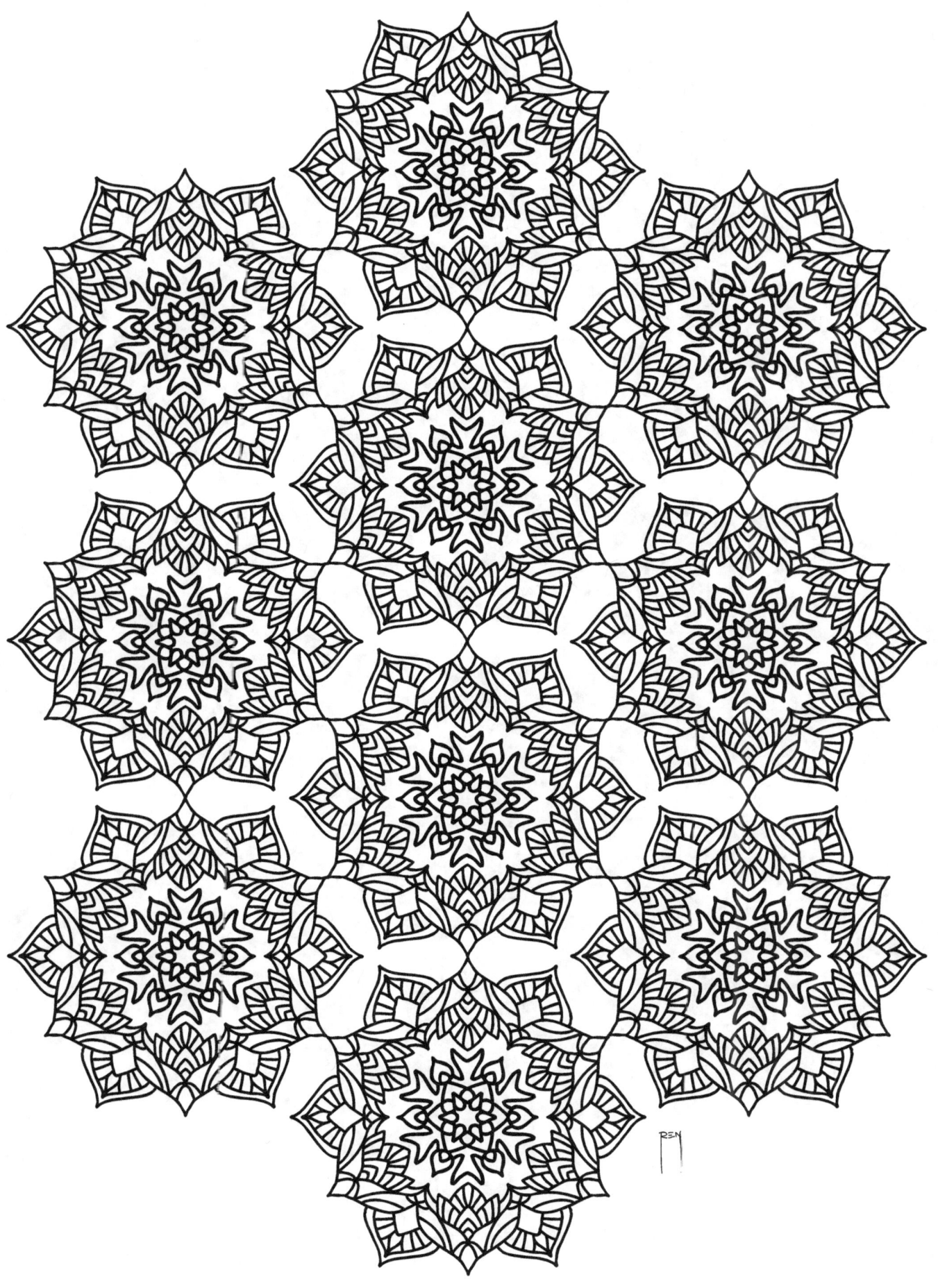

THE RECLAIMING OF MAGIC

Rejection of the Mundane

One of my favourite comments that some parents make about abstract art is: "My kid could do that!" And how right they are. The reason children are able to create rich, imaginative, and evocative imagery is because they are still drenched with magic. Their play is their work, and children take their work seriously.

As we get older, we allow our magic to slip away, to be left behind with our toys and games — the tools of the sacred work we once approached with such reverence. And we instead learn how to eat passionless food; watch countless hours of unexciting films, shows, and video clips; wear the clothes of nondescript people who want to look like everyone else; and we create art that has no Breath of Life, because we, ourselves, have been taught how to exist without Breath.

It's time to reclaim our magic, to breathe New Life into everything we do. It all starts with a little scribble. Go ahead and make a mark on this page, on any page, and scribble something frivolous, something nonsensical. It doesn't have to look like anything or symbolise anything; it only has to *be*. And then do it again. Once we learn to celebrate our scribbles, then we'll be worthy of our magic once again.

You are cherished.

Idea:
These designs can be incorporated into your quilt or other textile projects; search online for various methods to print or transfer images onto fabric

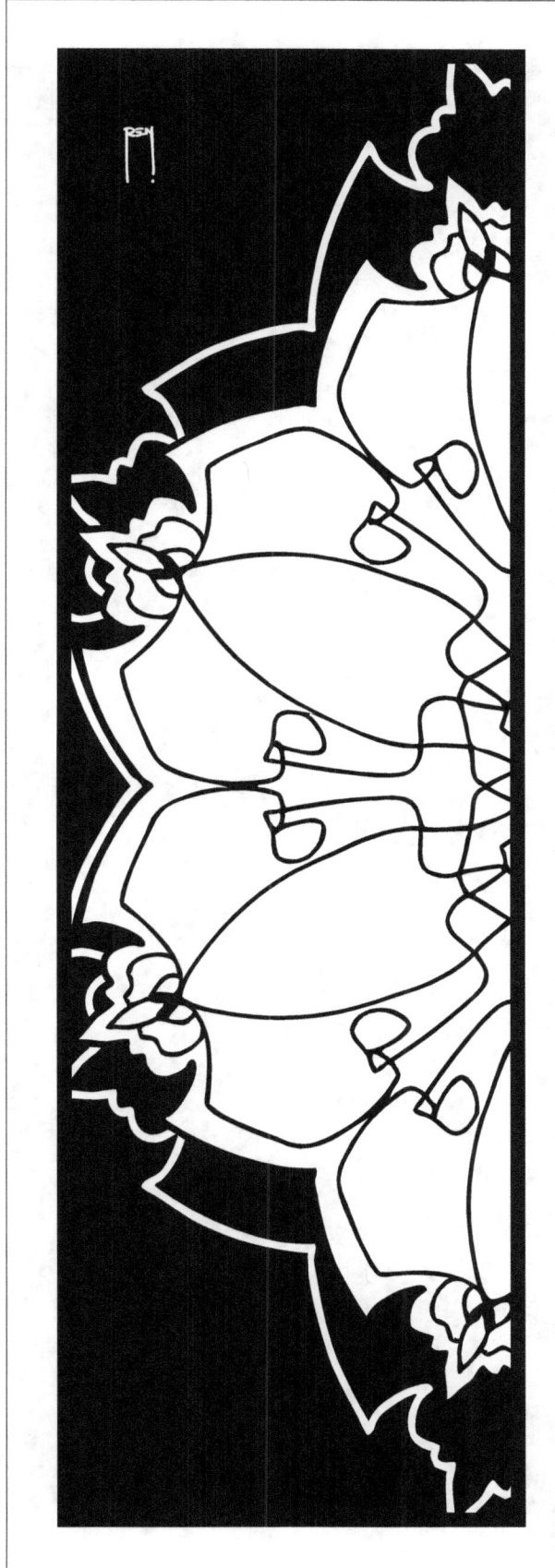
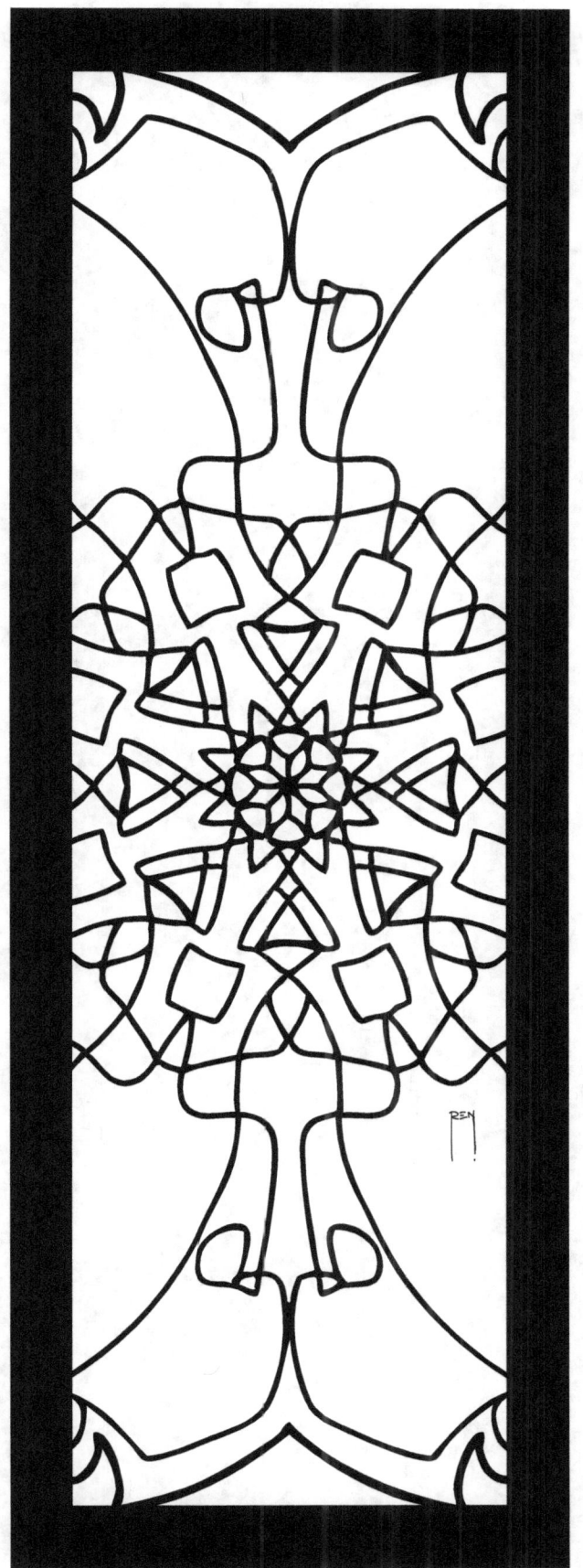

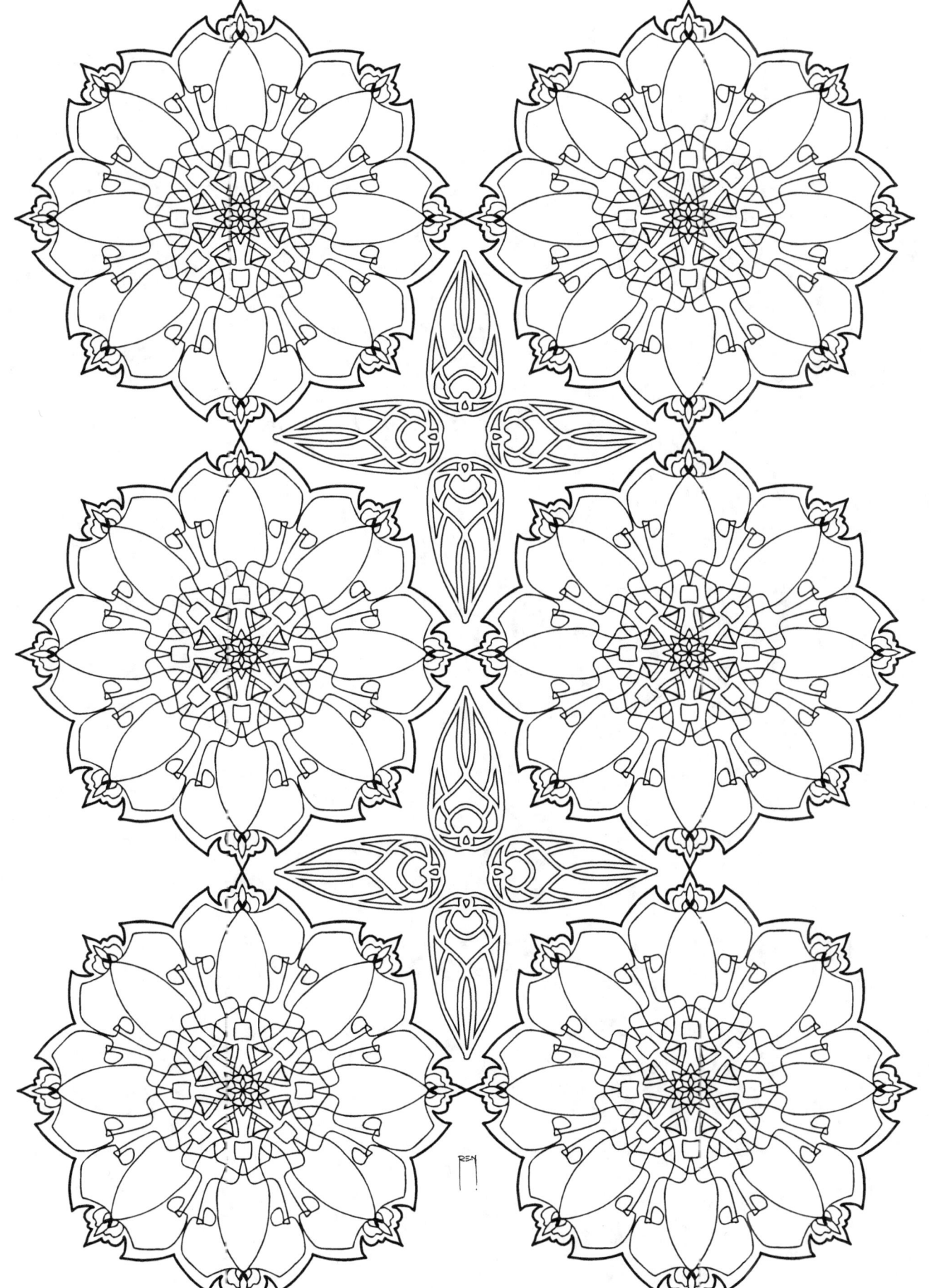

Idea: When fully coloured, slip these full-page pattern sheets under a glass table, dresser, or counter top to add instant visual interest

THE ALLURE OF HYPNOSIS

Captivation & Escape

During the two weeks I spent in the company of a great hypnotist, I was able to witness an intriguing aspect of the human psyche by observing as he worked. I came to the conclusion that people are drawn to hypnosis for two reasons: there is a thrill in the idea that one can be held captive by a charismatic stranger; and there is another,

paradoxical, thrill in the idea of escaping said stranger. When one is captive, one can be commanded to do a number of things that one normally wouldn't; and upon release of this immense power, one feels the rush of being "back to normal" in one's own mind.

The fascinating thing is that this "hold" over a person can only happen when one *allows* it to happen. We *invite* the hypnotist to captivate us, much like a child who delights in being discovered in a game of hide-and-seek. This hypnotist told me that people *allow themselves* to be hypnotised all the time: by what media they take in; by the words of the people around them; and by the words they tell themselves. People are often so afraid of their own power, they just give it away.

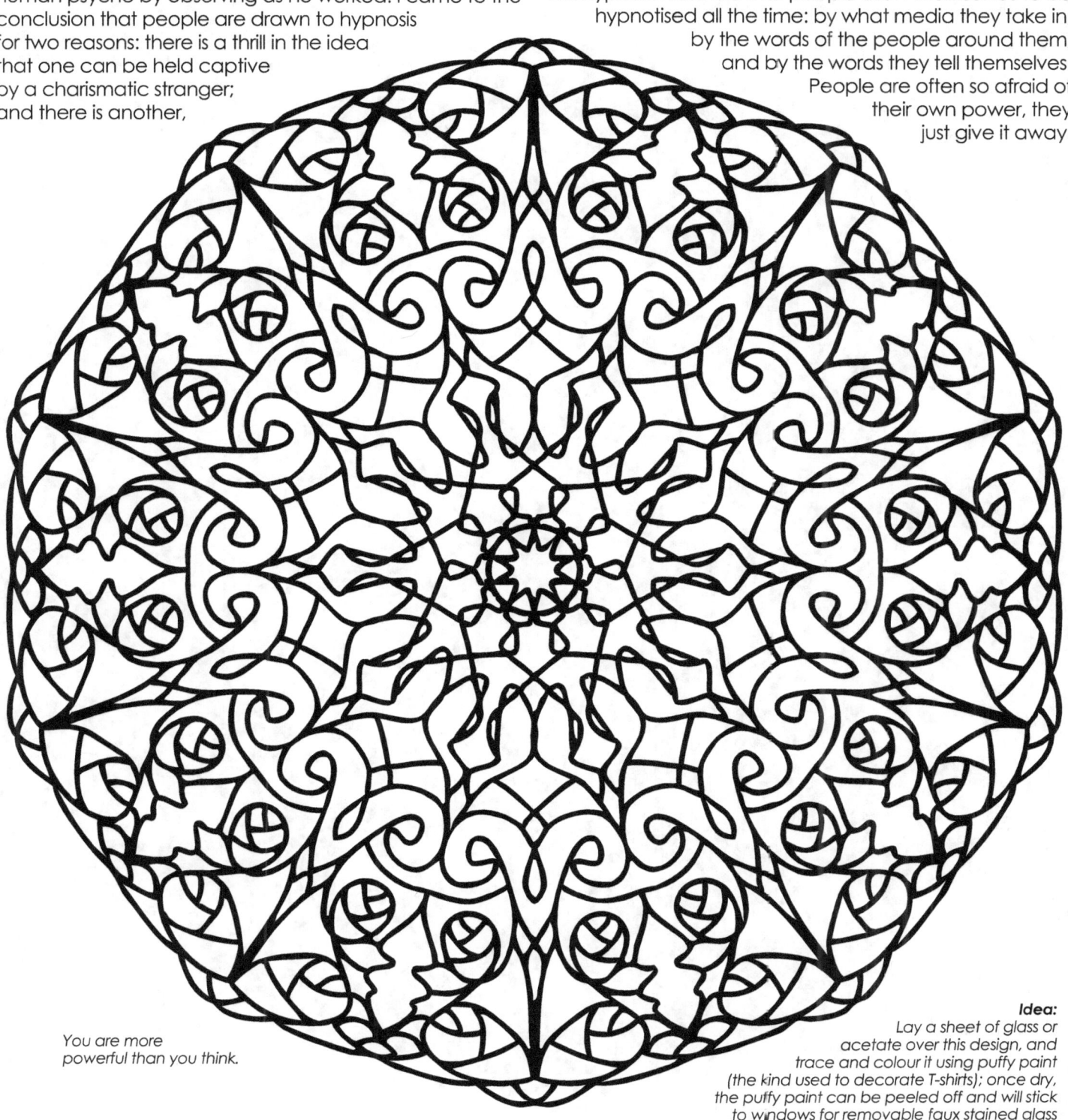

You are more powerful than you think.

Idea:
Lay a sheet of glass or acetate over this design, and trace and colour it using puffy paint (the kind used to decorate T-shirts); once dry, the puffy paint can be peeled off and will stick to windows for removable faux stained glass

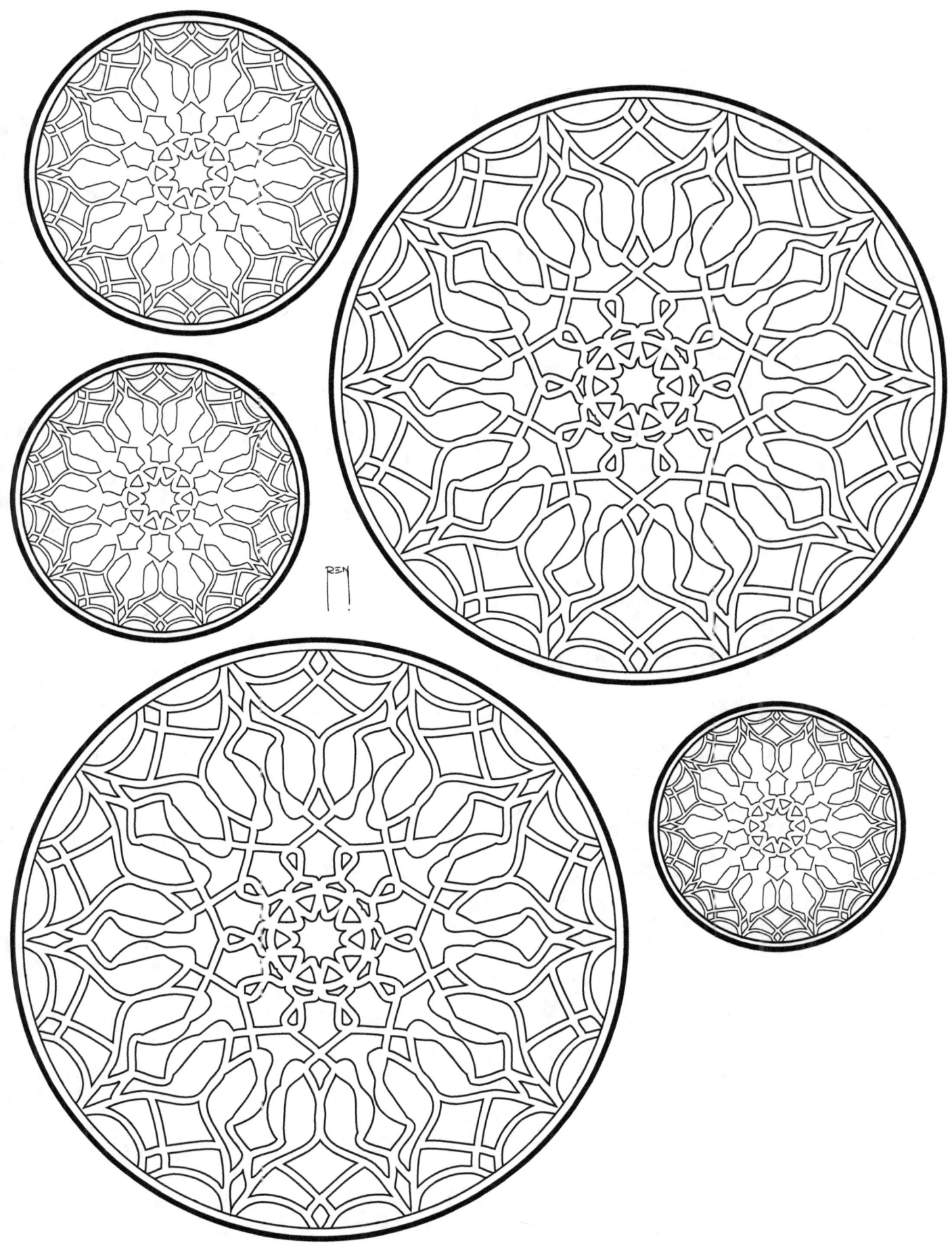

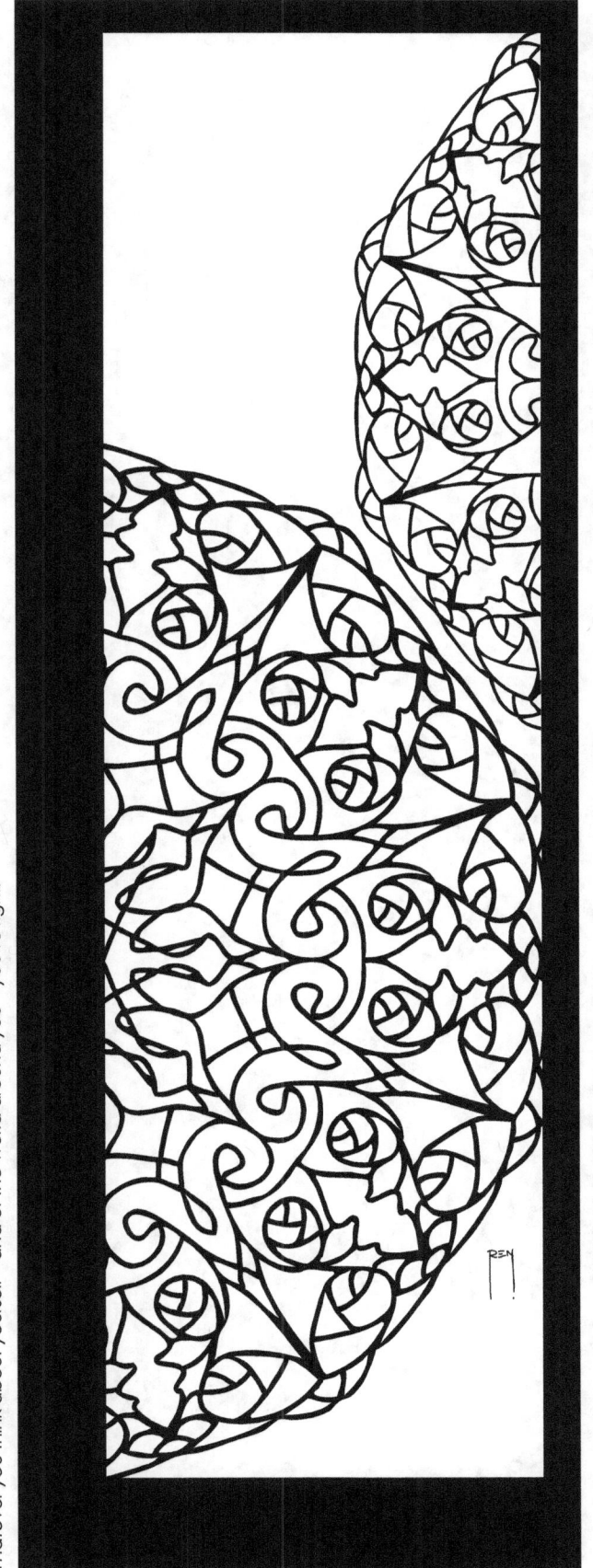

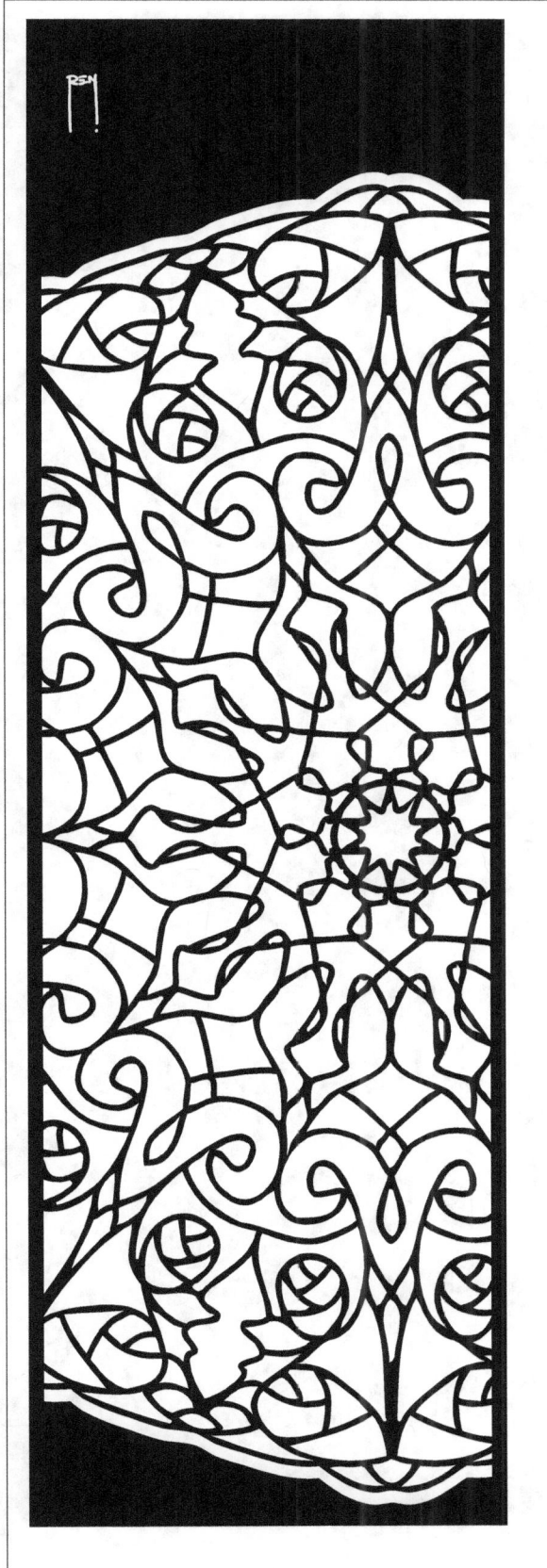

Whatever you think about yourself – and of the world around you – you're right.

Idea: Laminate these deigns so that you can colour them again and again with dry erase markers

THE IMMORTAL STRAND

A Taste of Forever

Imagine what it would be like to live a hundred years, or a thousand, or ten thousand. It's likely that our ancestors imagined this, too, or else we wouldn't have stories of gods and vampires.

Here's a different way of looking at it, from the perspective of the ancients: if they *had* entertained thoughts of immortality, then, through their strands of DNA that we possess, they do, in fact, still walk the earth, but with our bodies as their vessels. Perhaps even our intellect, instincts, and impulses are theirs as well; after all, studies have confirmed that much of our personalities are determined by our characteristics from birth — from nature, rather than nurtured. We would then be mere links in some very long chains of existence; we would be pieces of "forever."

If you did have a thousand years to live, what would you do with that time? If you have difficulty imagining this, think back on your life up to this point; what have you done with your current number of years? Now multiply it by twenty, fifty, or a hundred or more — how is your imagined millennium starting to look now?

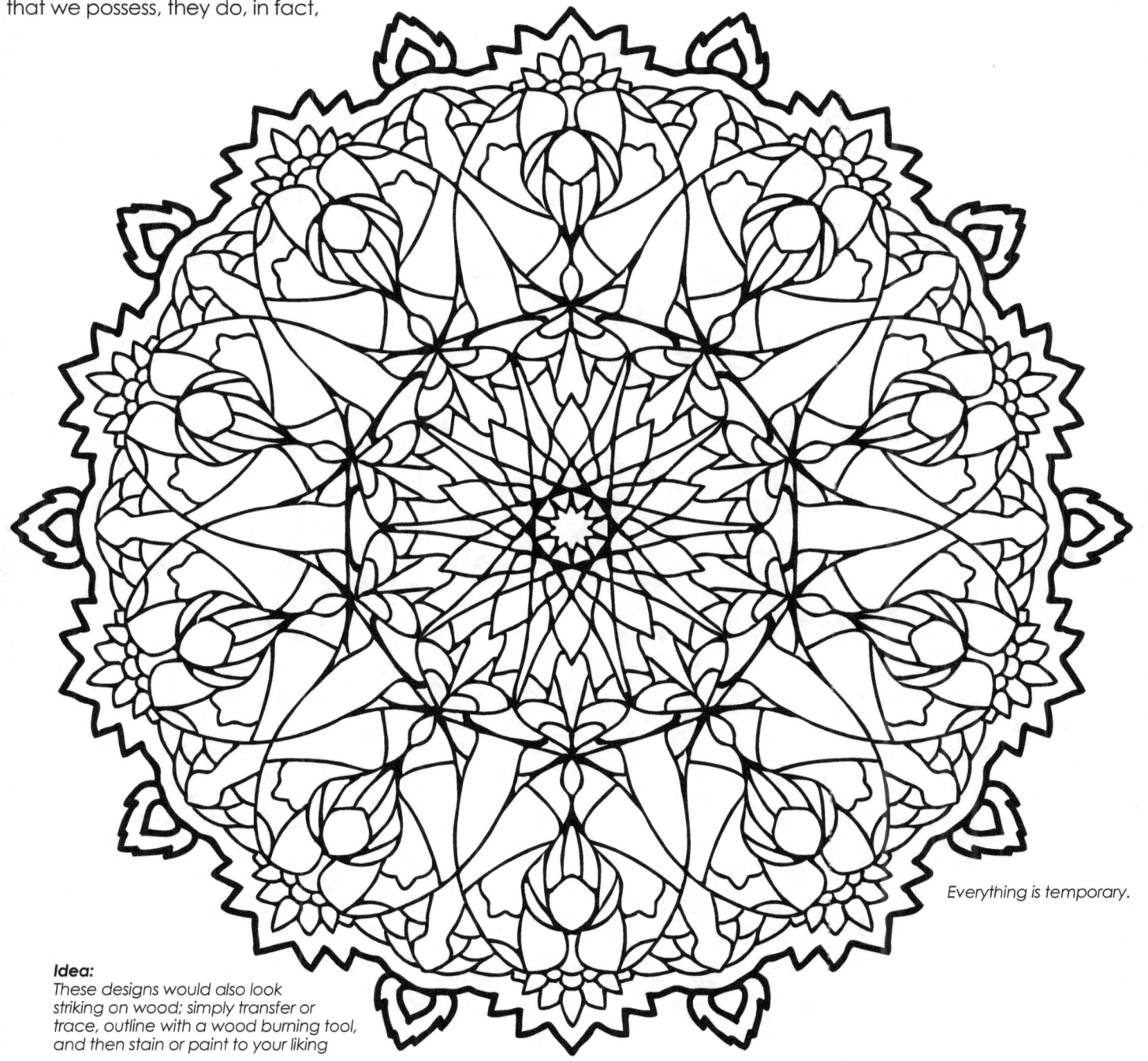

Everything is temporary.

Idea:
These designs would also look striking on wood; simply transfer or trace, outline with a wood burning tool, and then stain or paint to your liking

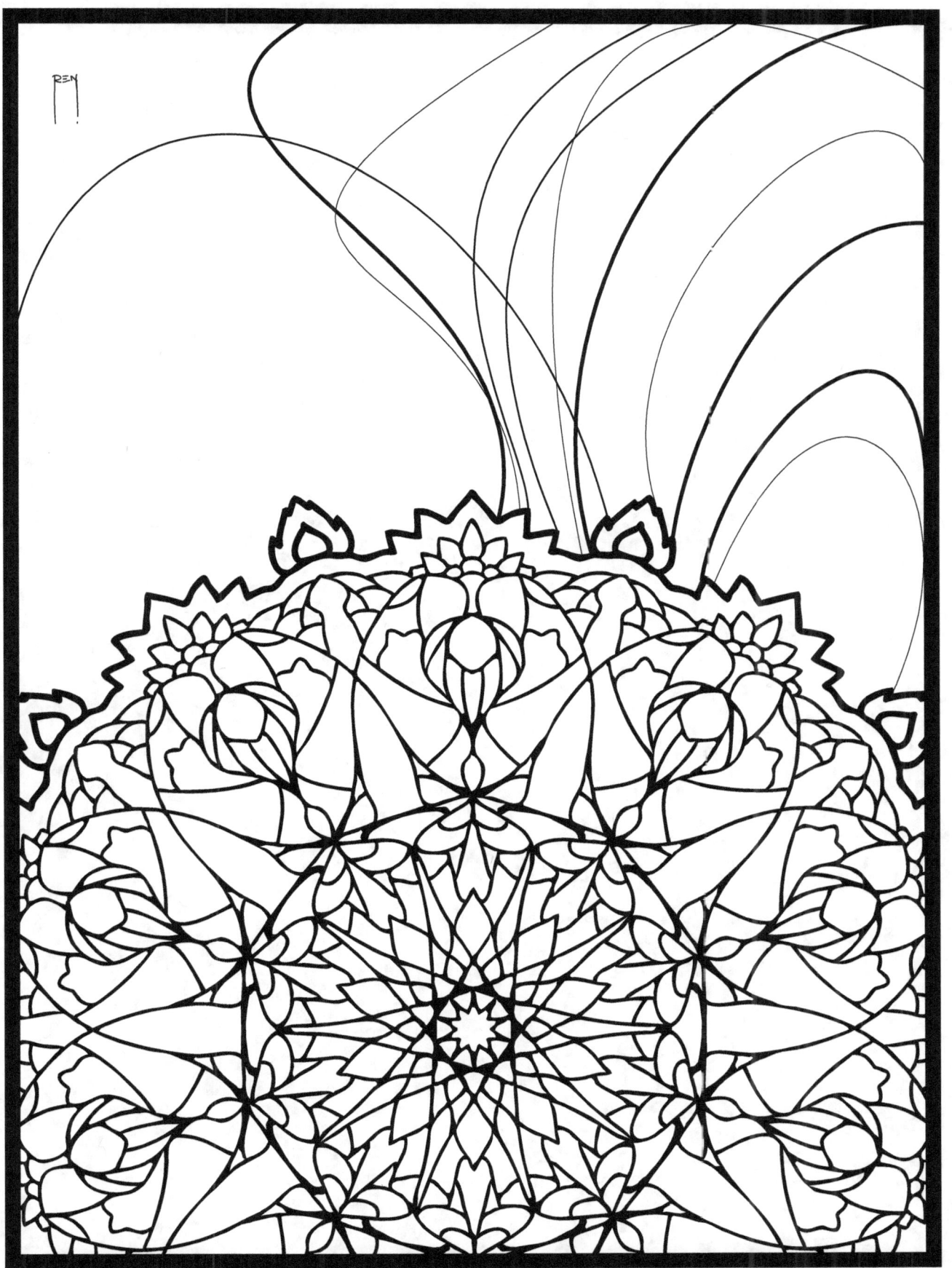

REN

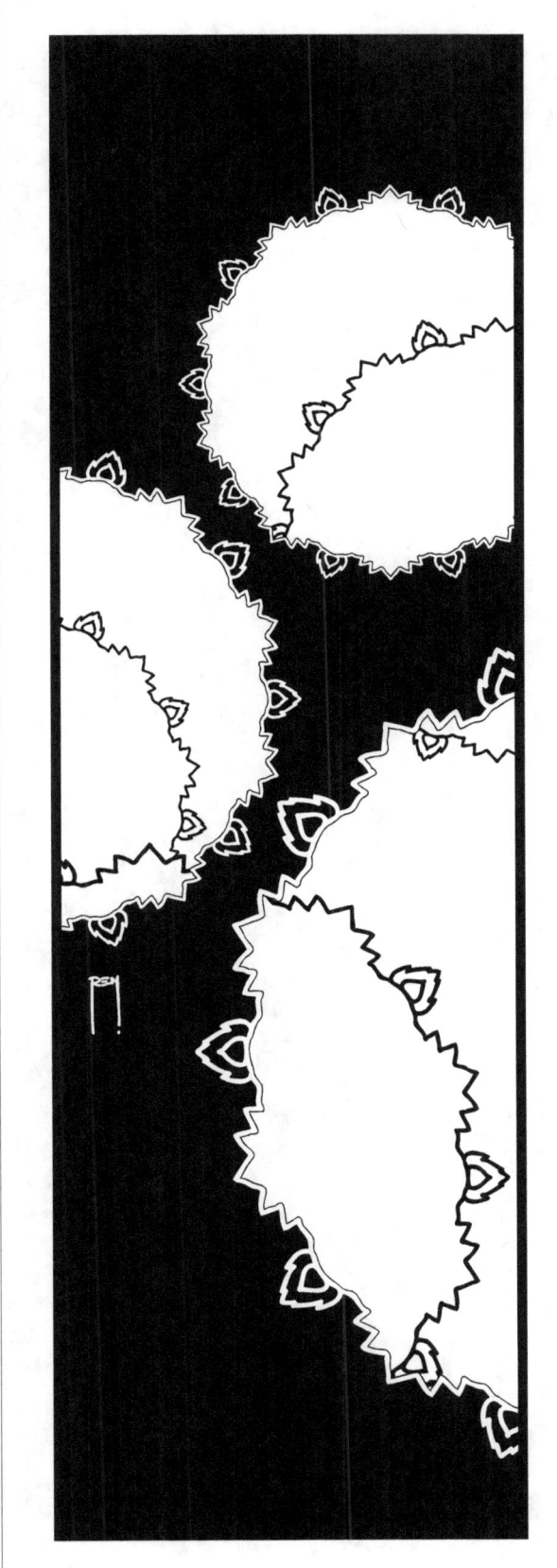
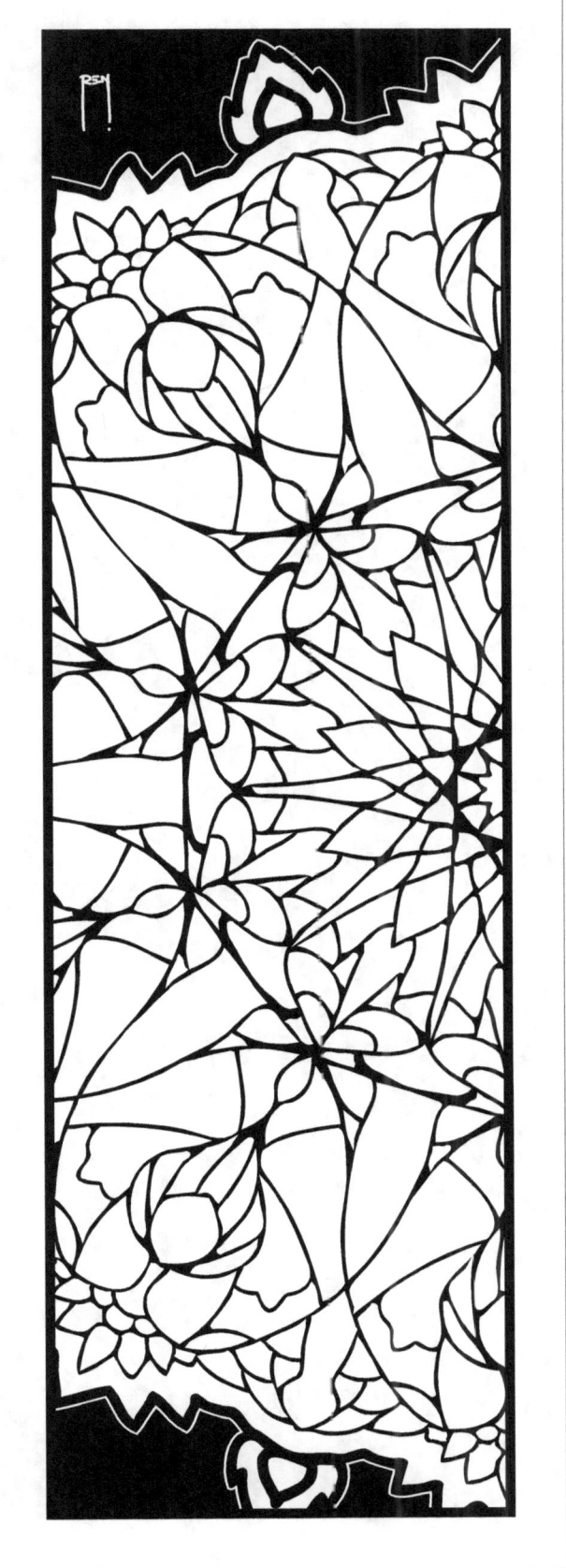

THE HUNDRED MUSES

Reflections of Endless Inspiration

The ancient Greeks had nine muses to provide guidance and inspiration for art, literature, music, and more. These nine muses were invoked before commencing one's creative work, to help guide the mind, body, and spirit on the right path to bring the work to fruition.

In the commercial art world, there's no such thing as "waiting for inspiration," and we often need a great deal of help to remain productive and prevent burnout. So, while students at art university, a friend and I came up with *The Hundred Muses*, sources we identified within the self, as well as the world around us, which help nourish and encourage creativity.

Think about the many aspects of your personality, the facets you intensify or diminish (whether consciously or unconsciously) throughout your life. Give names to these aspects, and when you need them — for example, the part of you called "The Great Healer" — then you can invoke it by focusing on its name and qualities before undergoing any task or situation. This kind of mental exercise helps to promote mindfulness, which opens one's awareness to the present. For more about the Hundred Muses, look for our series, *Master Mandalas: The Hundred Muses*.

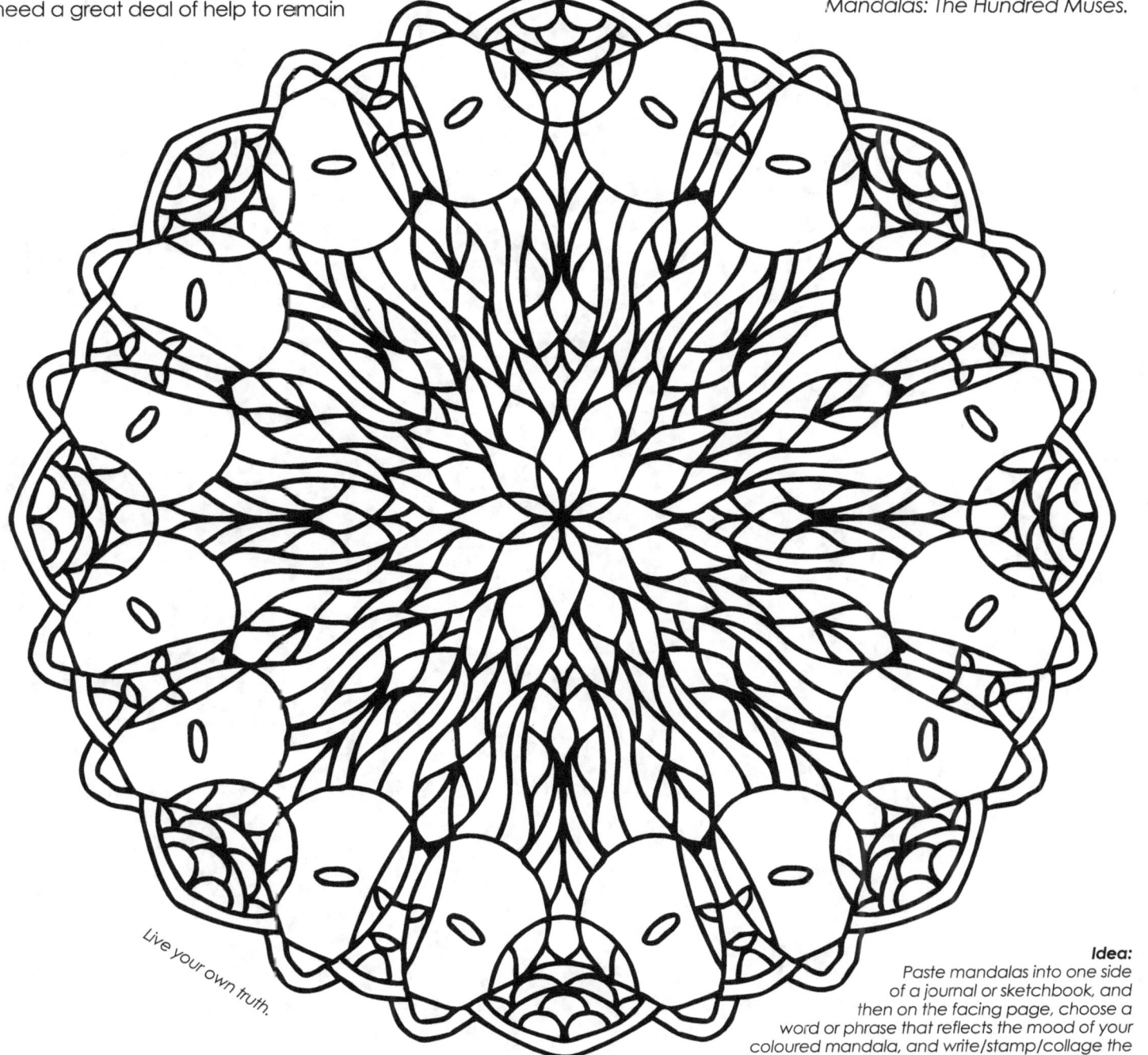

Live your own truth.

Idea:
Paste mandalas into one side of a journal or sketchbook, and then on the facing page, choose a word or phrase that reflects the mood of your coloured mandala, and write/stamp/collage the word or phrase in a decorative or meaningful way

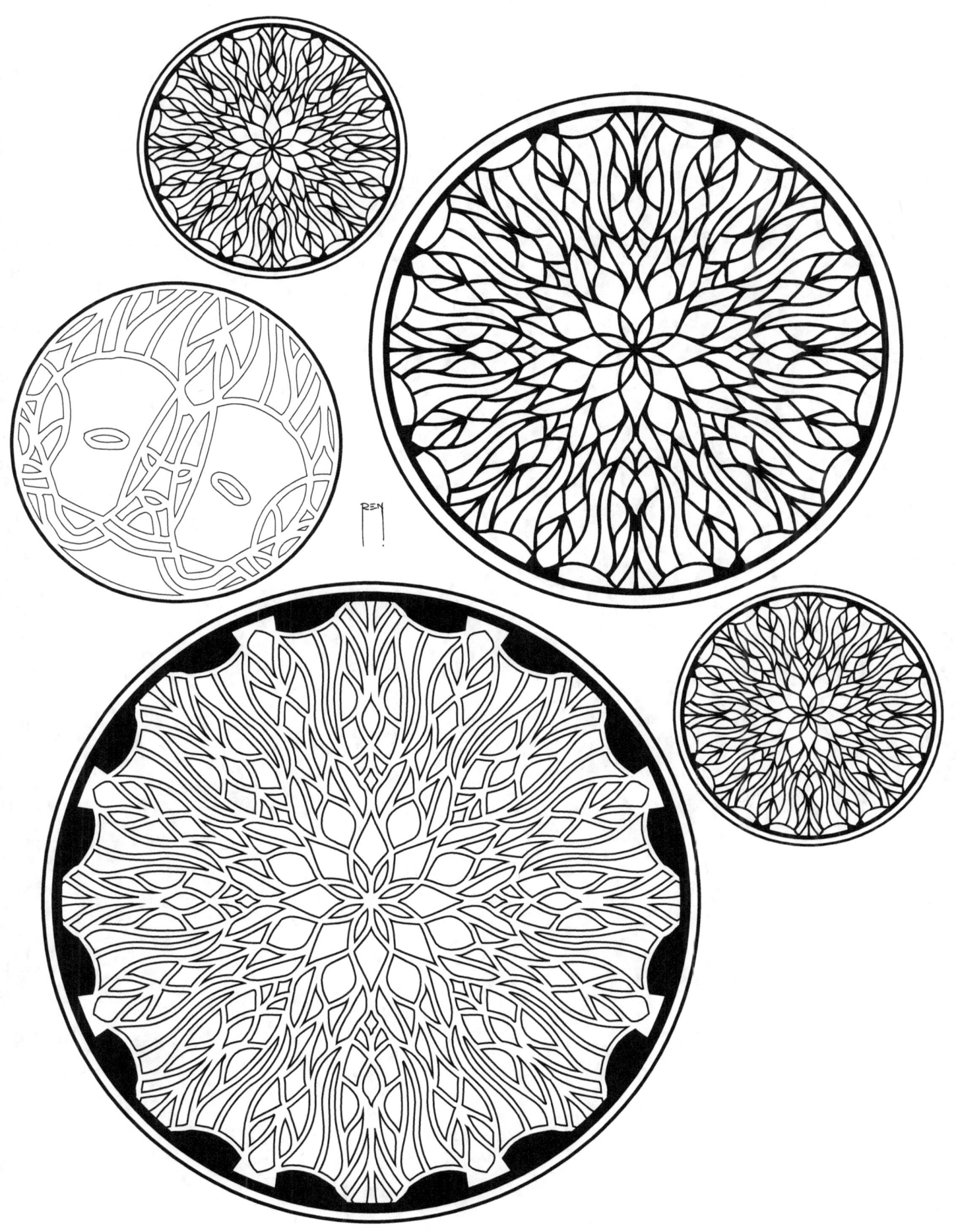

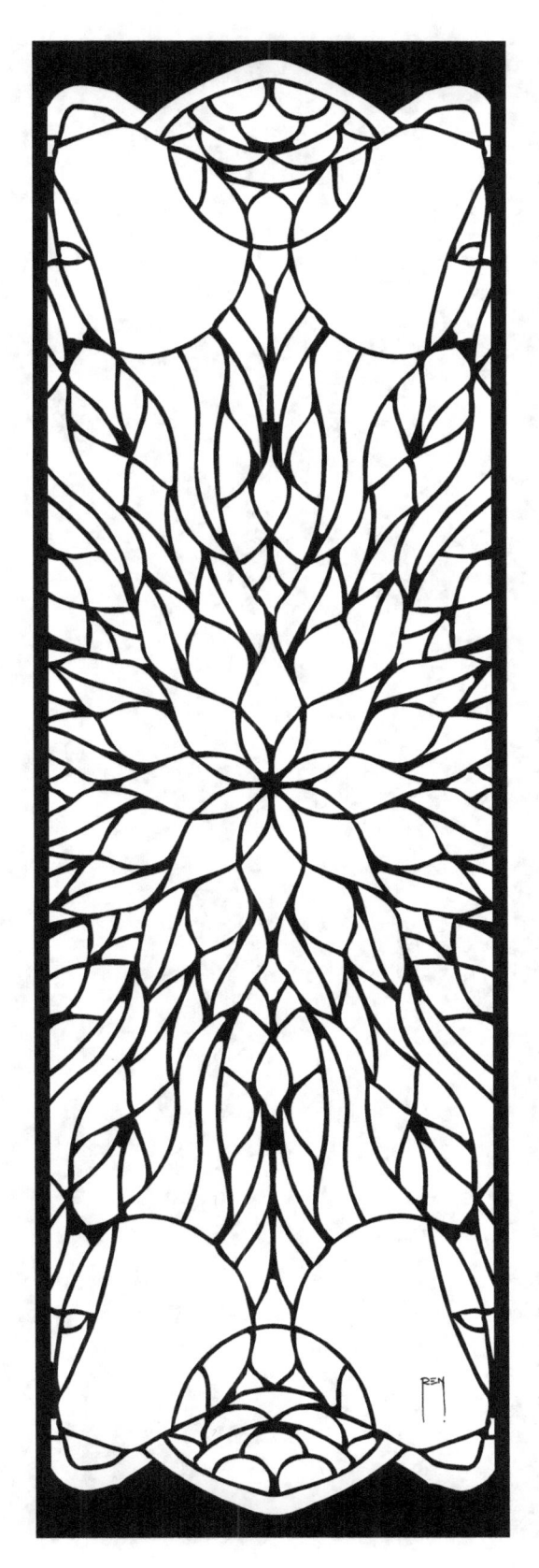

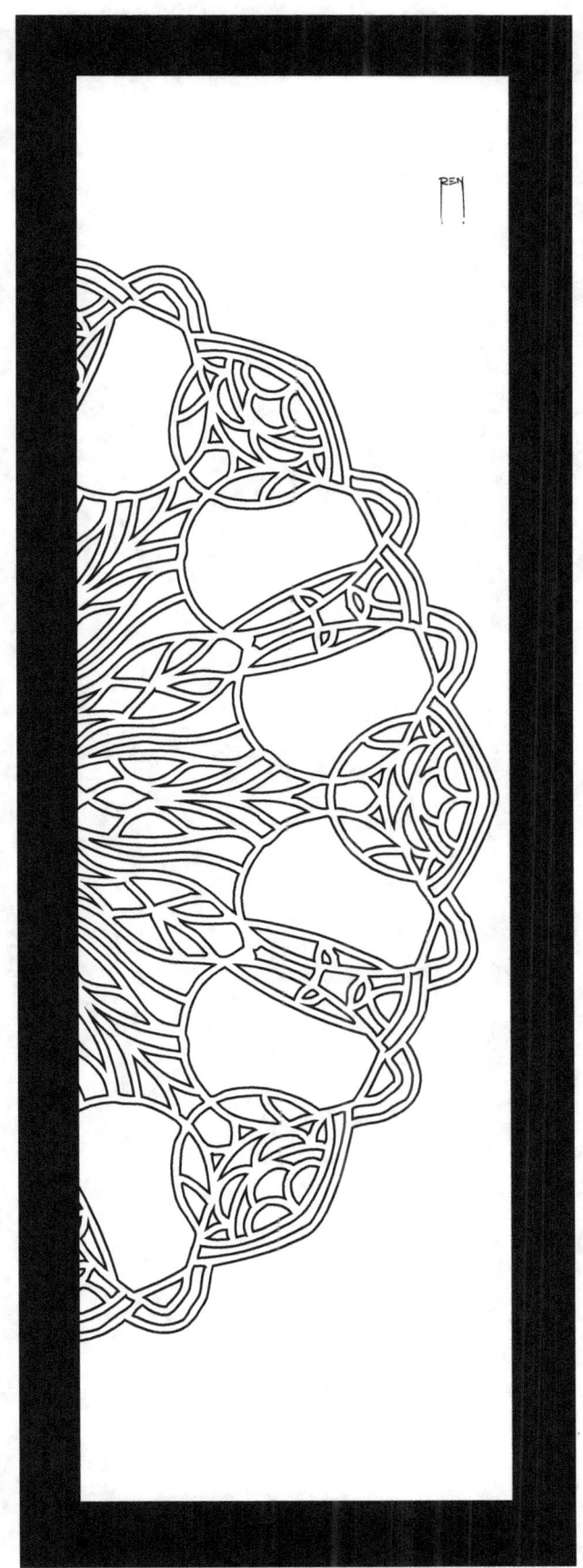

Growth and change are often painful. Pain is merely weakness leaving the body.

THE LIVING LIBRARY

The Most Valuable Books in Existence

In many societies throughout history, elders have been revered for their wisdom and experience. They carry the stories of their ancestors, as well those of their children, and perhaps even their children's children. Elders encourage ritual and culture; they provide insight, hindsight, and serve to expand the perspectives of the young; they were Google before there was Google. Their value is immeasurable, and their firsthand accounts of historical events — told in their own words, voices, and facial expressions —

will always have greater impact and meaning than any wiki article could convey. Each person is a book, and the most fortunate are the ones who have amassed chapters and stories that can entertain, teach, and touch the heart.

When you think about your life in terms of stories and chapters, what are the "pages" — the anecdotes, the special moments — that stand out to you? If you feel that your life book is lacking, then you can add richness by incorporating the knowledge and lessons from the elders in your life. Talk with them; ask them questions; and allow their stories to add depth to your own. Think of it as adding a prologue or footnotes to your book of life. As you collect stories, write them down or record them on video or audio for posterity.

Idea:
Colour and laminate these designs to use as doilies under a candy dish; glue onto card stock for added strength

You are deserving of love; you always have been, and you always will be.

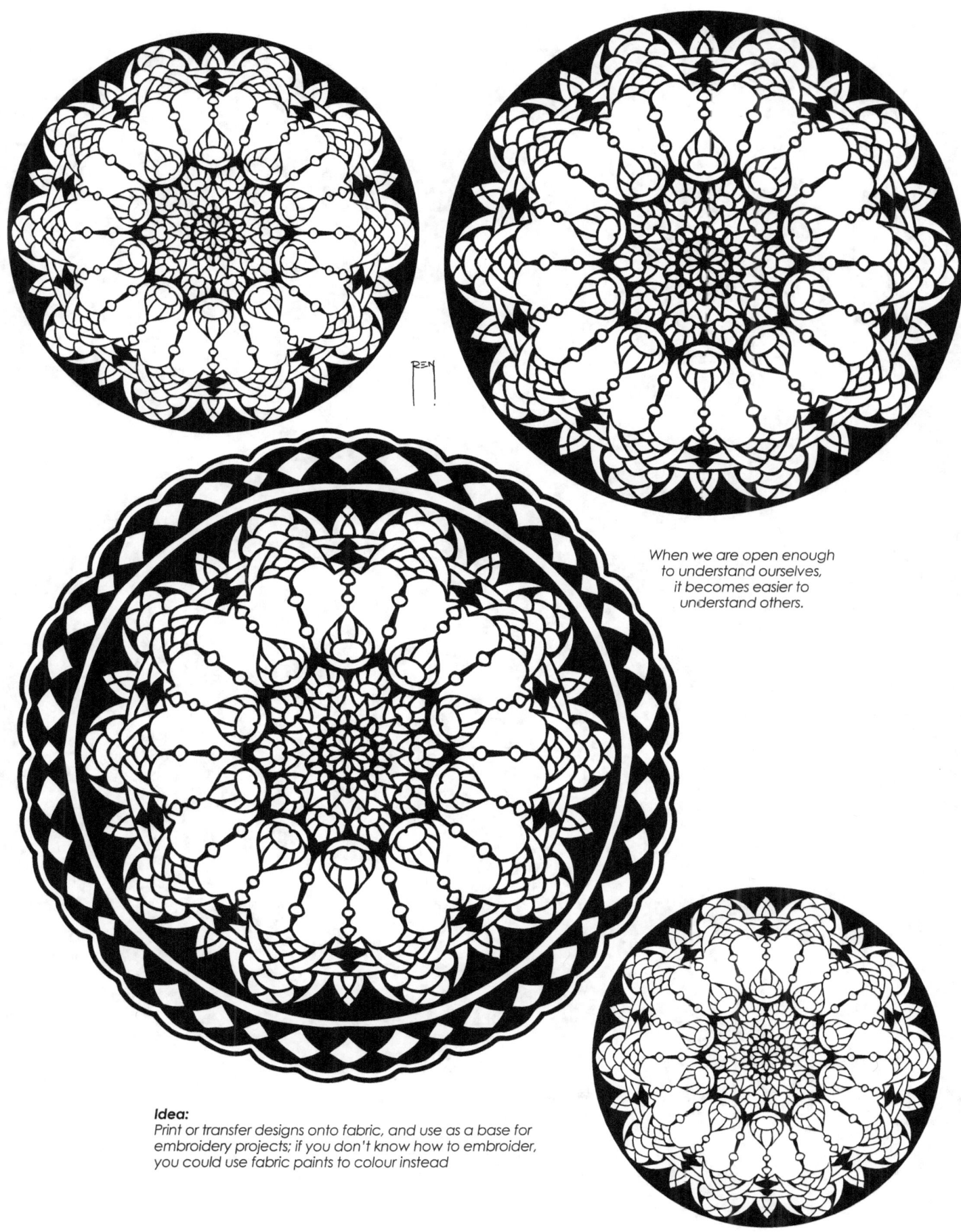

When we are open enough to understand ourselves, it becomes easier to understand others.

Idea:
Print or transfer designs onto fabric, and use as a base for embroidery projects; if you don't know how to embroider, you could use fabric paints to colour instead

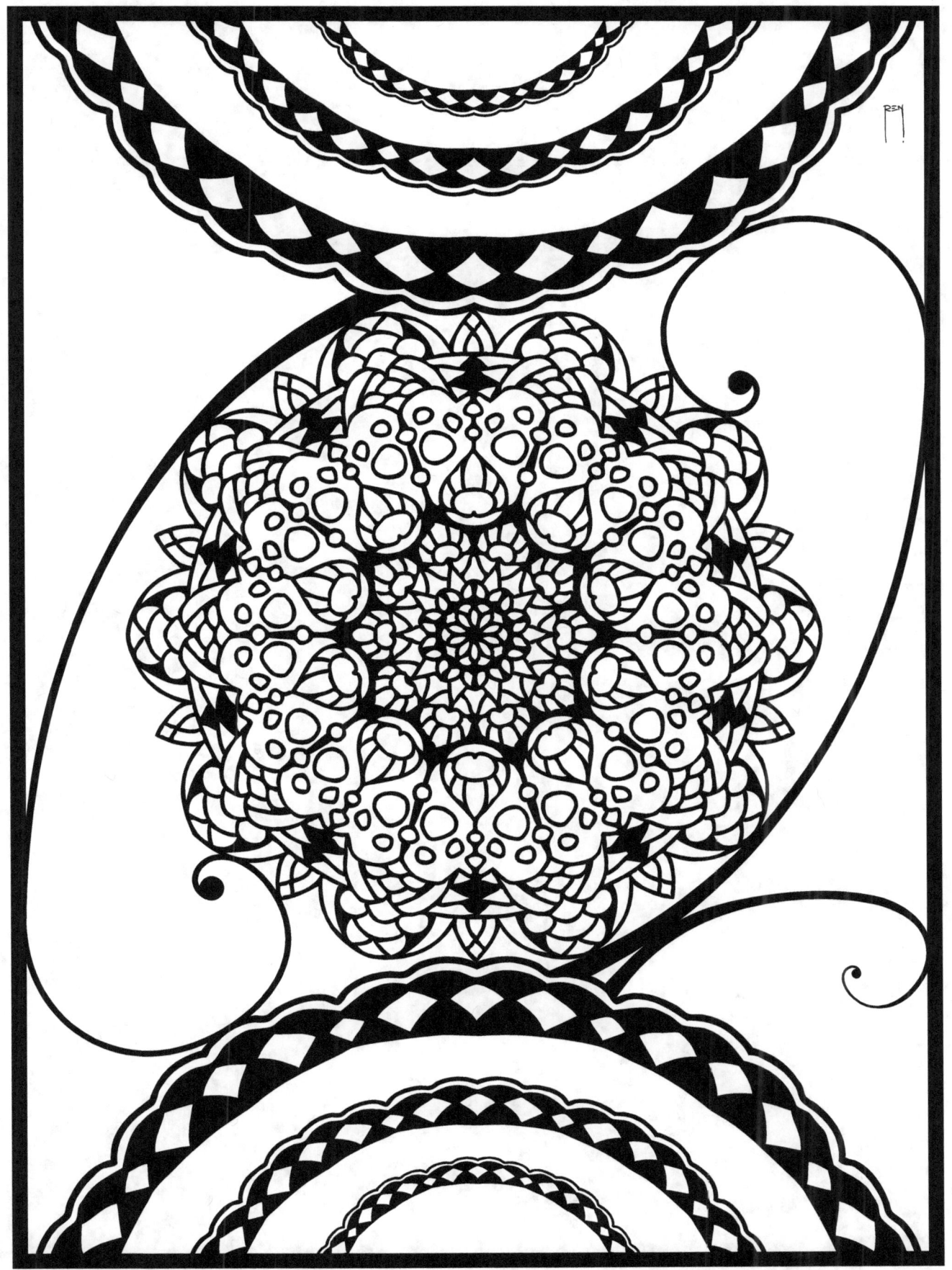

THE MAGIC OF WORDS

Every Breath is a Spell Cast

In the Hawaiian culture, we believe that spoken words have power; they are magical, and anything that is spoken, uttered, or even whispered contains *mana*, a concept of life energy that is similar to the Asian belief in *chi* (or *qi*). Mana can be transferred through speech, hence the importance of prayer, chants, and song. Because of this belief, many Hawaiians will not address their friends and loved ones in derogatory terms, a departure from mainland American popular culture, in which profane words — or even "softer" insults, such as "dummy" — are often used as an accepted way of expressing closeness with one's friends.

Imagine that your words are mystical, that the longings and wishes you speak will somehow come true. What are some of the things you would wish for yourself or those close to you? Speak the words to create the magic.

Imagine the path of your life from this point forward; see and feel the choices you will make, the people you will meet, the things you will accomplish. Speak of them aloud, as though your words are a spell that you cast over yourself. What kinds of wonders await you?

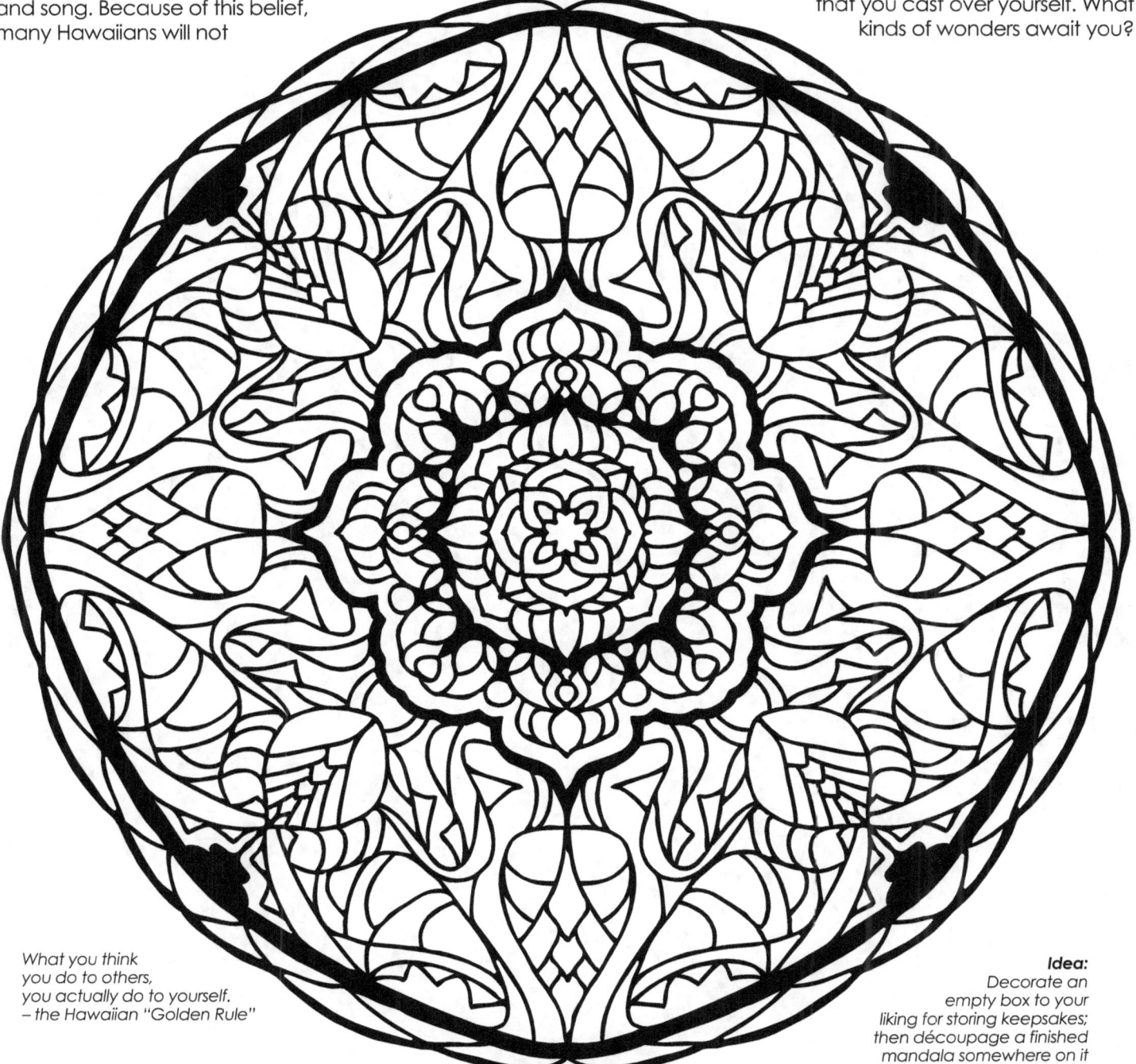

*What you think
you do to others,
you actually do to yourself.
– the Hawaiian "Golden Rule"*

Idea:
*Decorate an
empty box to your
liking for storing keepsakes;
then découpage a finished
mandala somewhere on it
for a striking focal point*

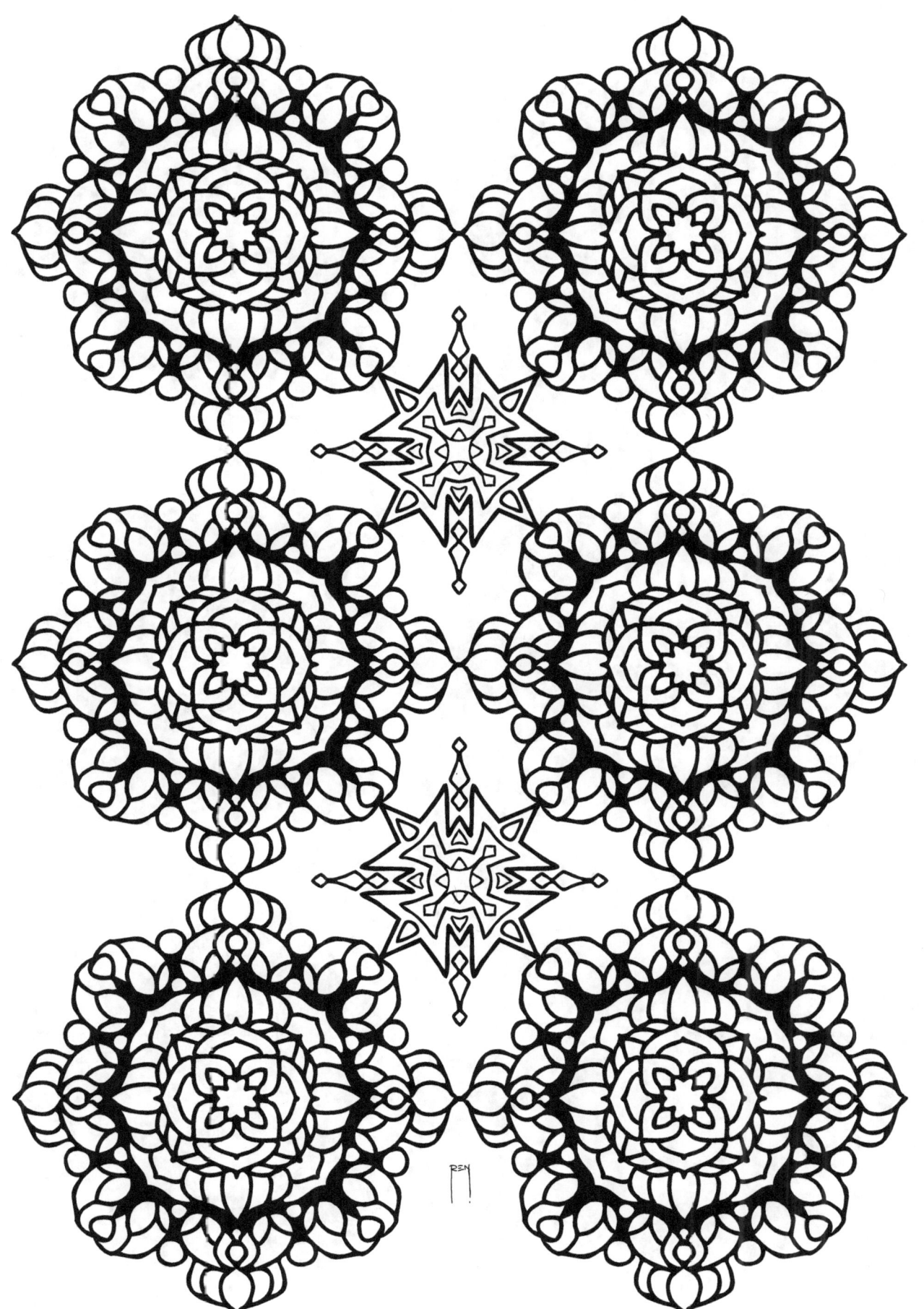

Sometimes we have to ask for help, and that's okay. It doesn't mean that we're weak; it means that we're human.

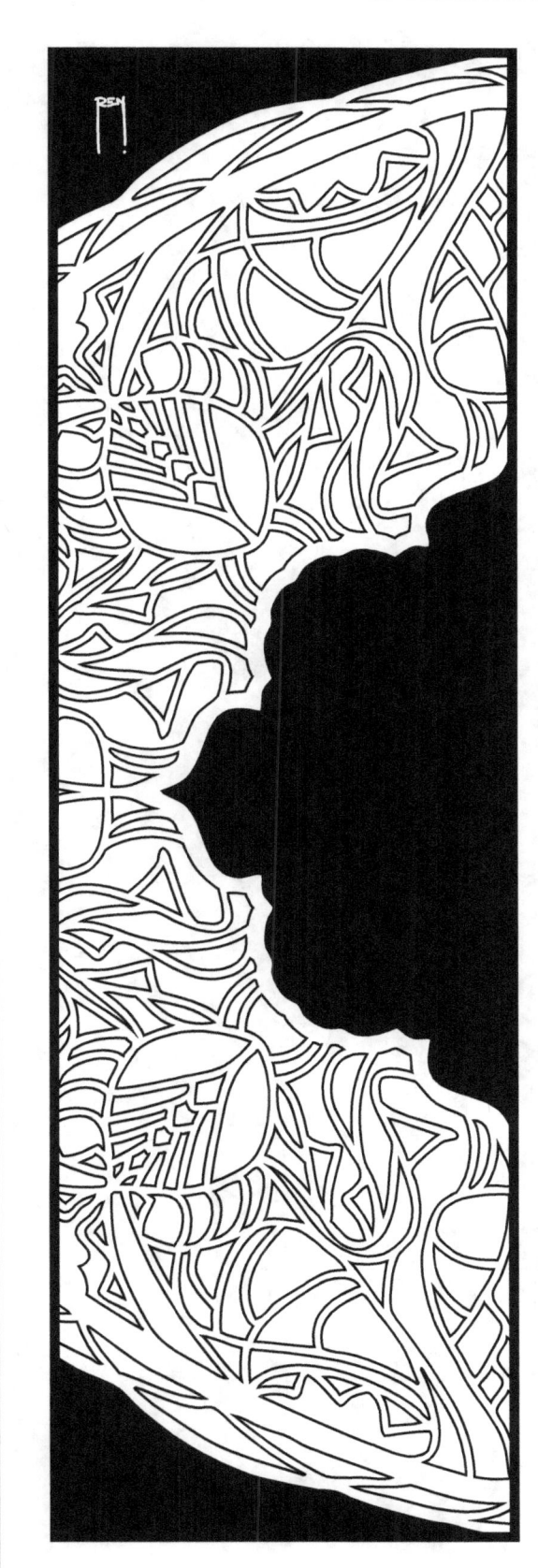

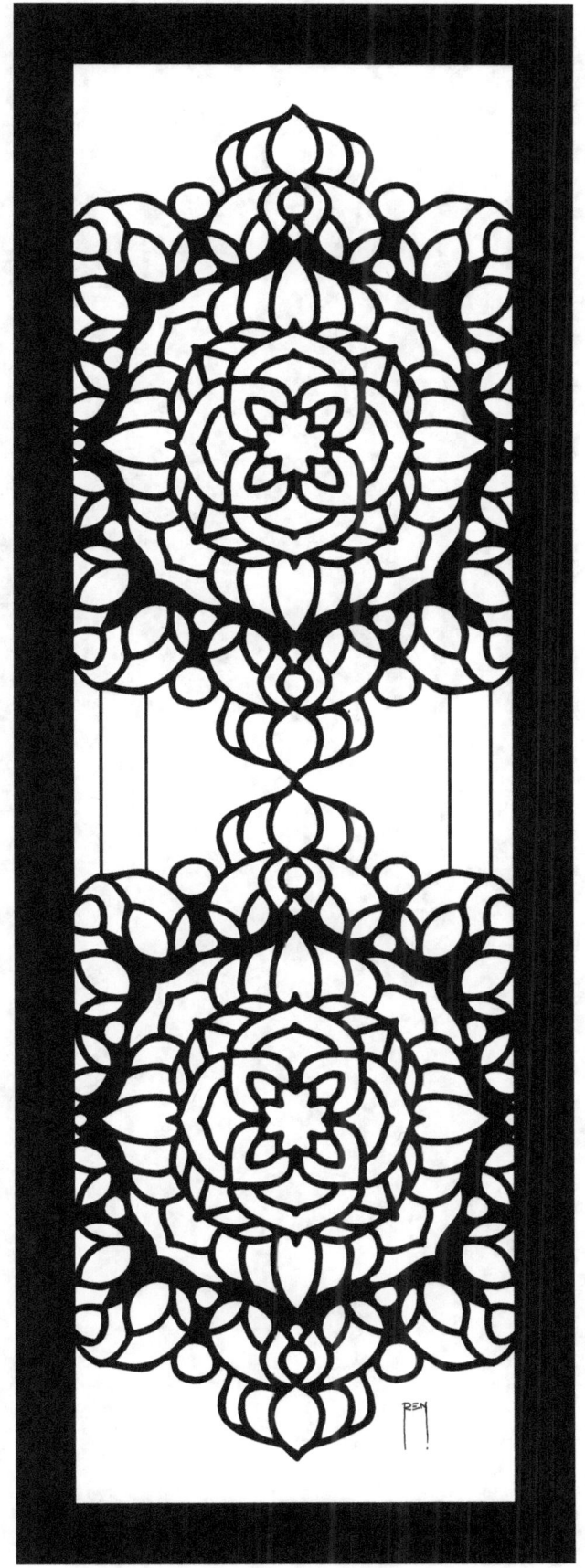

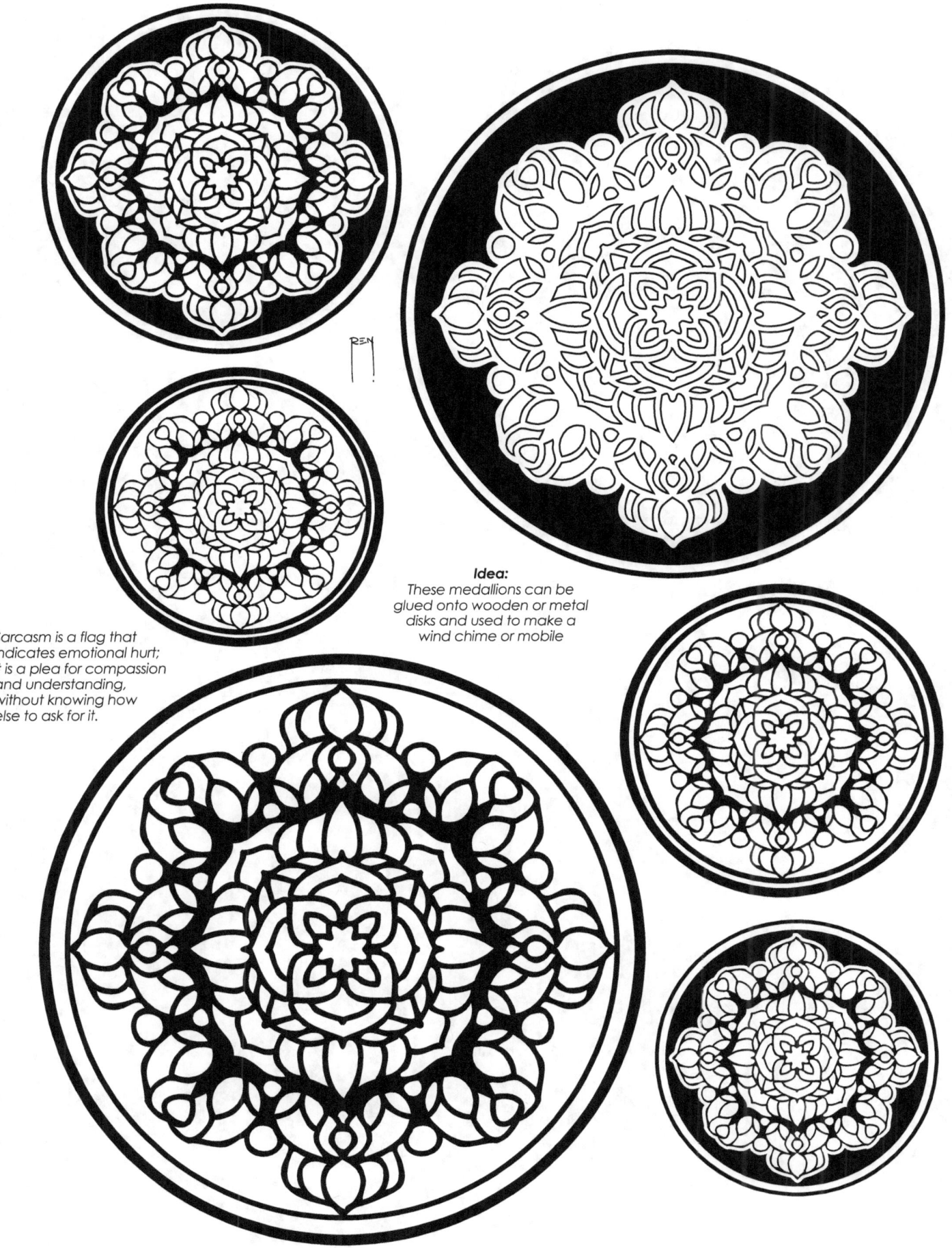

Idea:
These medallions can be glued onto wooden or metal disks and used to make a wind chime or mobile

Sarcasm is a flag that indicates emotional hurt; it is a plea for compassion and understanding, without knowing how else to ask for it.

The Strength of Softness

Sensitivity is a Powerful Force

The ancient Chinese martial arts masters enhanced their skills by observing the plants that surrounded them, the animals that lived among the plants, and the seasons that shaped the behaviour of the animals. From this observation, they learnt that the most resilient plants and animals possessed the qualities of softness, suppleness, and sensitivity. Bamboo that sways with the winds can survive storms, whereas trees can snap like toothpicks in a hurricane or monsoon. Likewise, being able to roll with literal punches helps disperse the force of the blow.

Some misunderstand the concepts of softness and sensitivity to mean weak and timid. This is not the case. The quiet strength contained within sensitivity is easily overlooked by those who seek explosive results. But for situations that call for elegant force, understanding your softness can be a powerful way to catalyse change.

One way to sharpen your emotional awareness is through journaling. Keep a record of the things that trigger emotional responses, and then write down your responses, thoughts, and actions. When you read through old journal entries, you'll be able to assess situations and determine how much, or how little, sensitivity would have been needed to obtain a positive or desirable outcome.

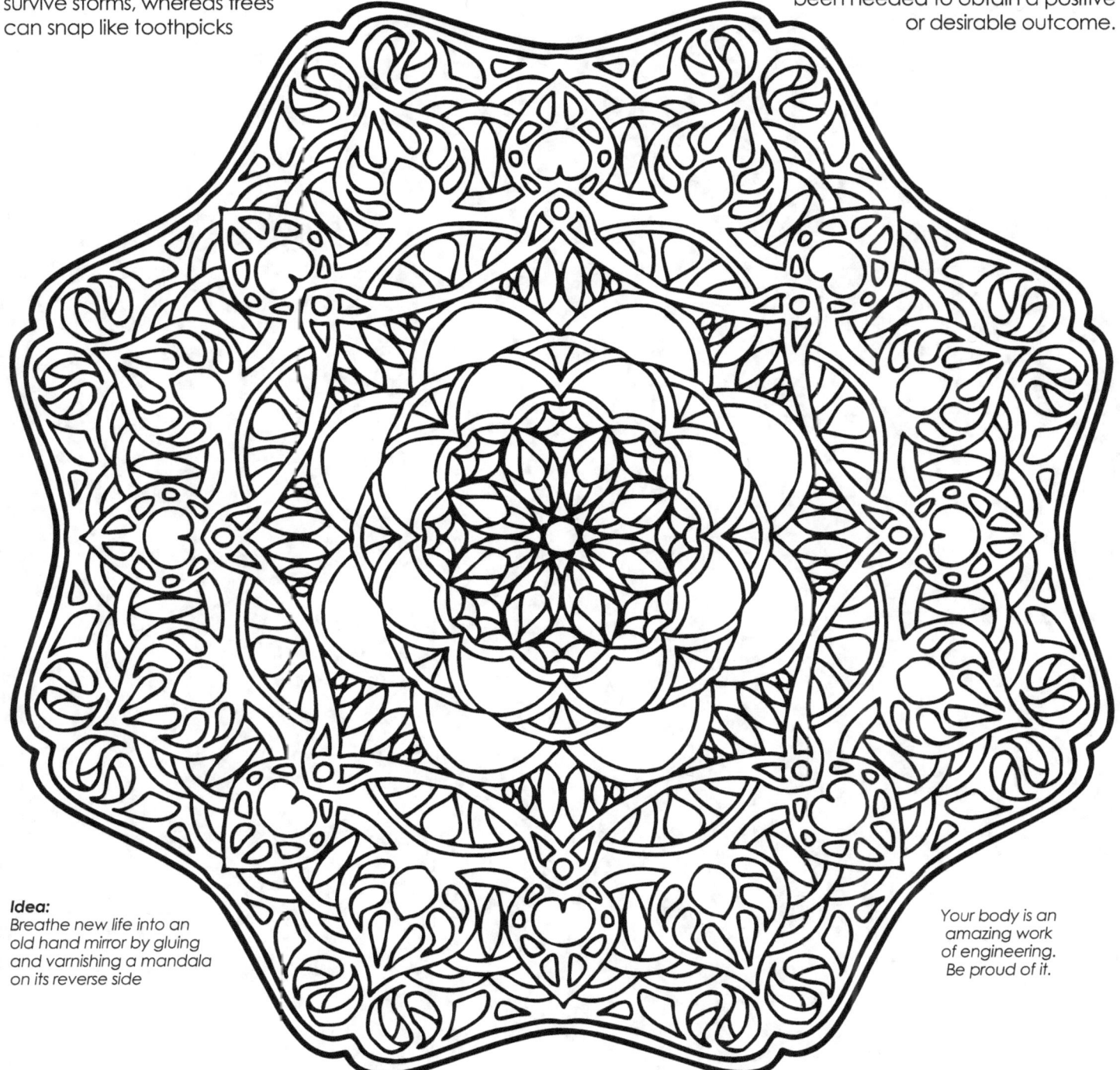

Idea:
Breathe new life into an old hand mirror by gluing and varnishing a mandala on its reverse side

Your body is an amazing work of engineering. Be proud of it.

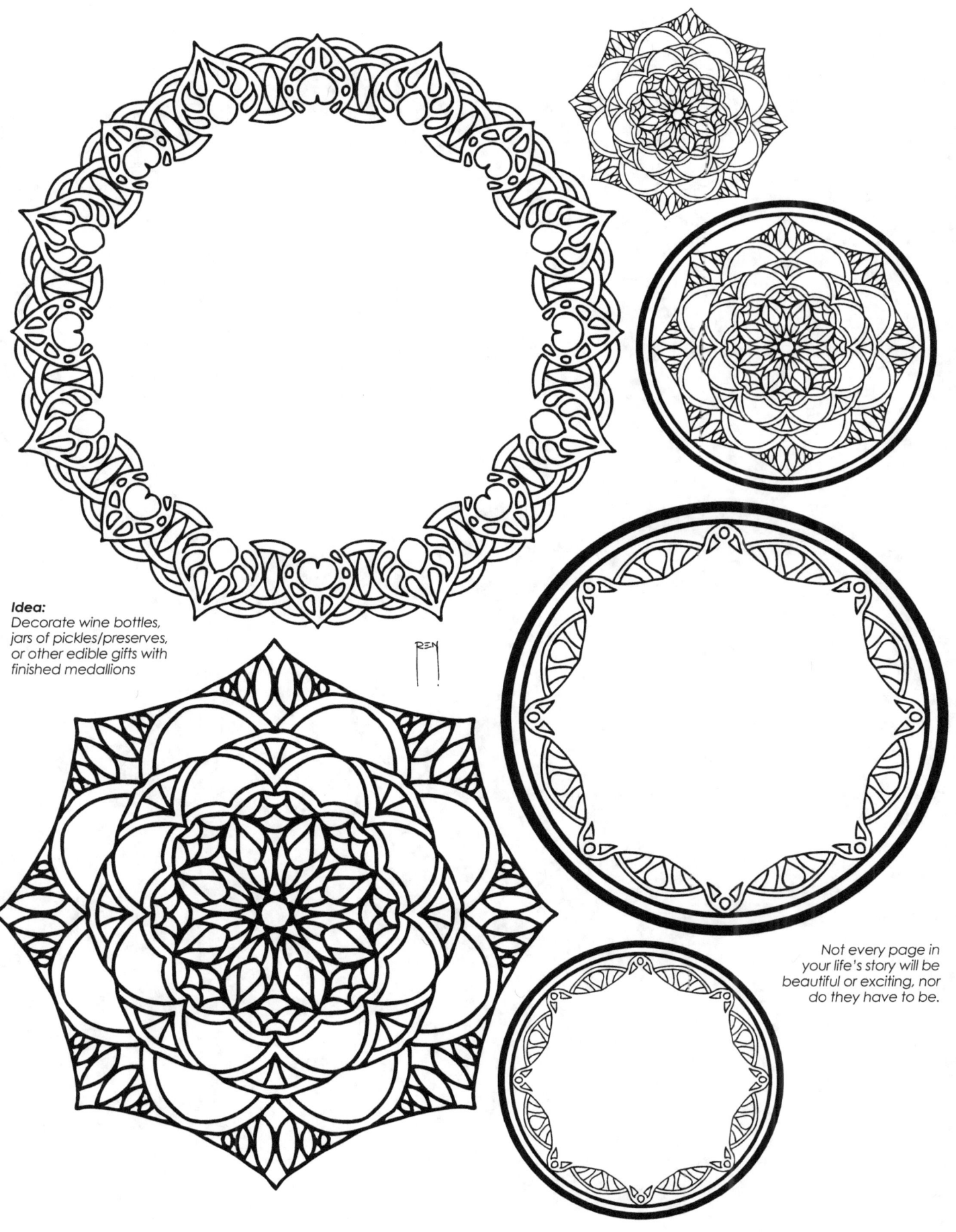

Idea:
Decorate wine bottles, jars of pickles/preserves, or other edible gifts with finished medallions

REN

Not every page in your life's story will be beautiful or exciting, nor do they have to be.

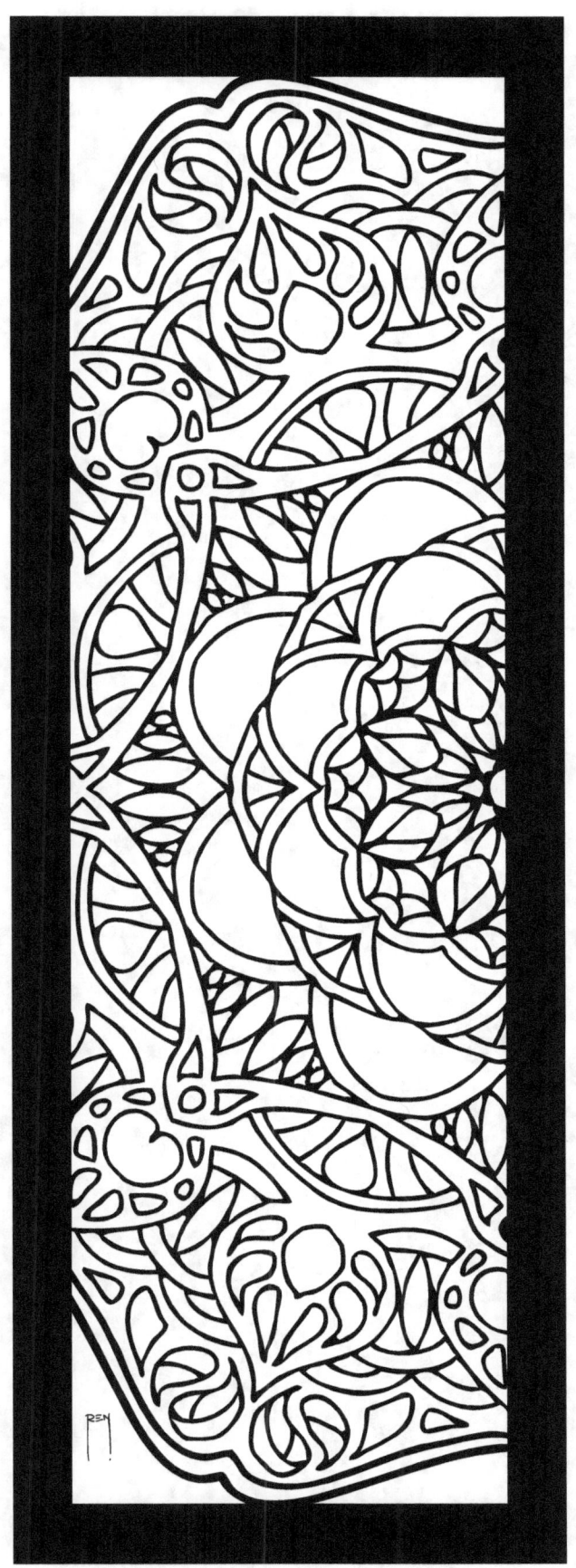

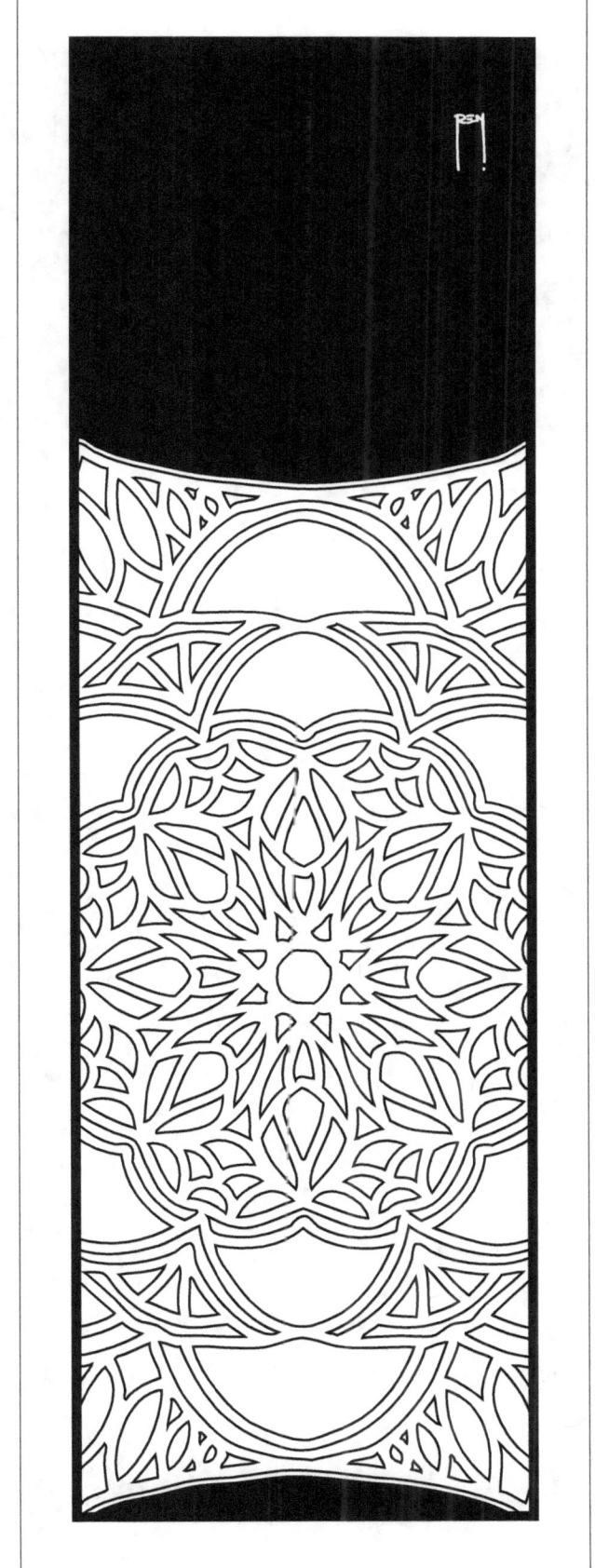

It is better to be soft, like water, than unyielding, like a rock; water can shape the rock or swallow it whole; there is power in being soft.

Idea: Cut out these bookmarks to add to your travelling artist's kit for colouring on the go

PULSE OF THE SUBCONSCIOUS

The Beauty of the Beast

When I was first introduced to the idea of the subconscious, I imagined it as a huge, dark purple kraken, an enormous, long-tentacled sea creature that lurked in the blackest depths of the mind. It was a mysterious and wild, untamable beast that was better left alone.

As I grew older and explored the subconscious, I learnt how to harness its immense power. I saw and felt its sublime beauty. And I witnessed its effects in my work.

The best way to deepen your creative well is to take in lots of references: read more literature and poetry; look at more paintings and sculptures; listen to music and watch films that challenge the way you think and perceive the world. The more you take in diverse and rich media, the more massive your creative well becomes.

If you are able, remove yourself temporarily from social media, phones, computers, and other technology for one day each week; if you can detach from technology for more than one day at a time, then that's even better. This "quiet time" will train you to listen to your subconscious mind, as well as allow you time for meditation or quiet reflection. Sometimes, personifying your subconscious makes it easier to get to know. If your subconscious were a beast or creature, what would it be, and how would it look?

You are a force of nature.

Idea:
Glue a mandala to the outside of a sealed envelope for a memorable piece of mail art that will delight the recipient

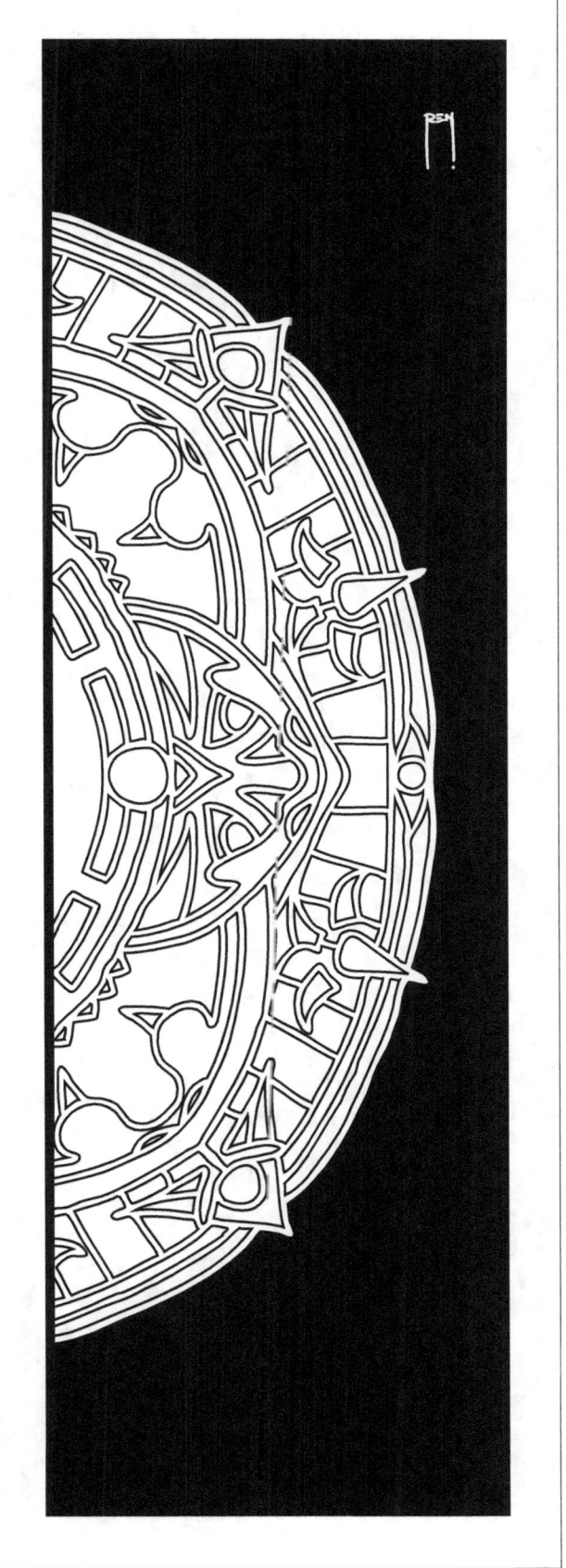

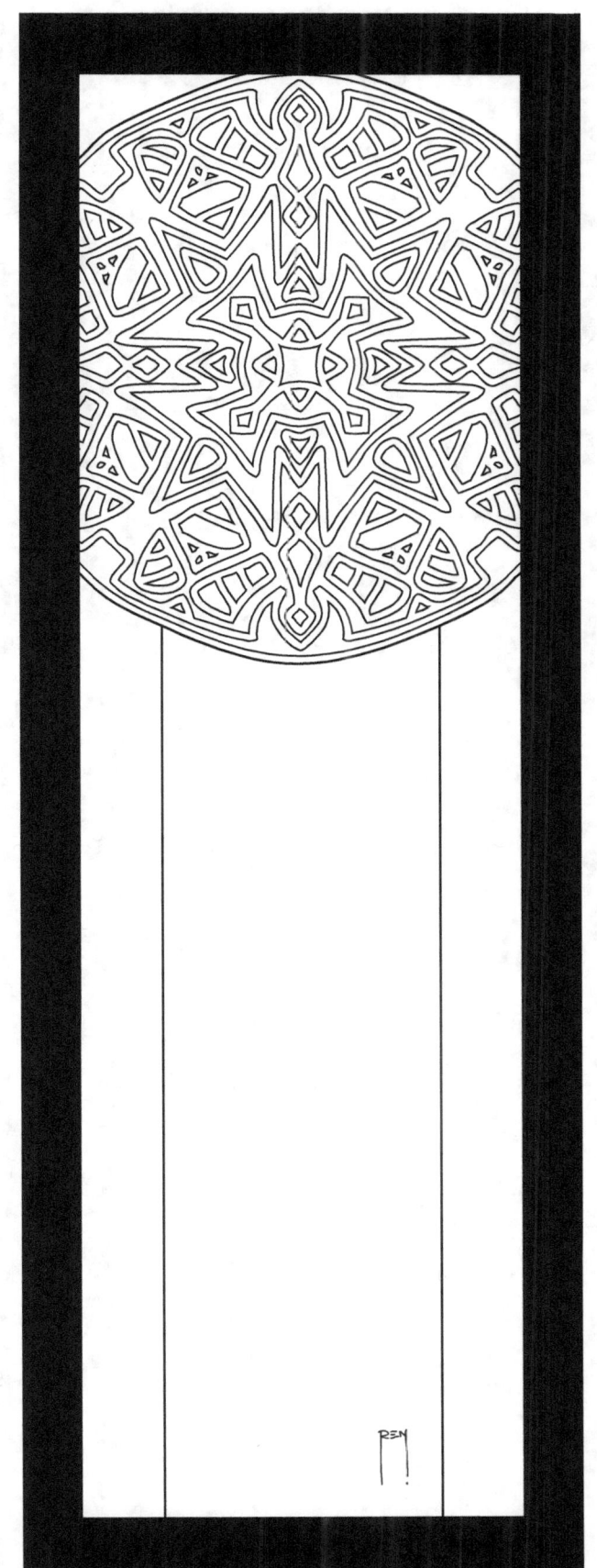

Idea: *These bookmarks can also be used as scrolls; write a message on the back, then roll it up, and secure with a rubber band, string, ribbon, or yarn*

Allow yourself five to ten minutes each day for total silence, including silencing your thoughts and inner voice.

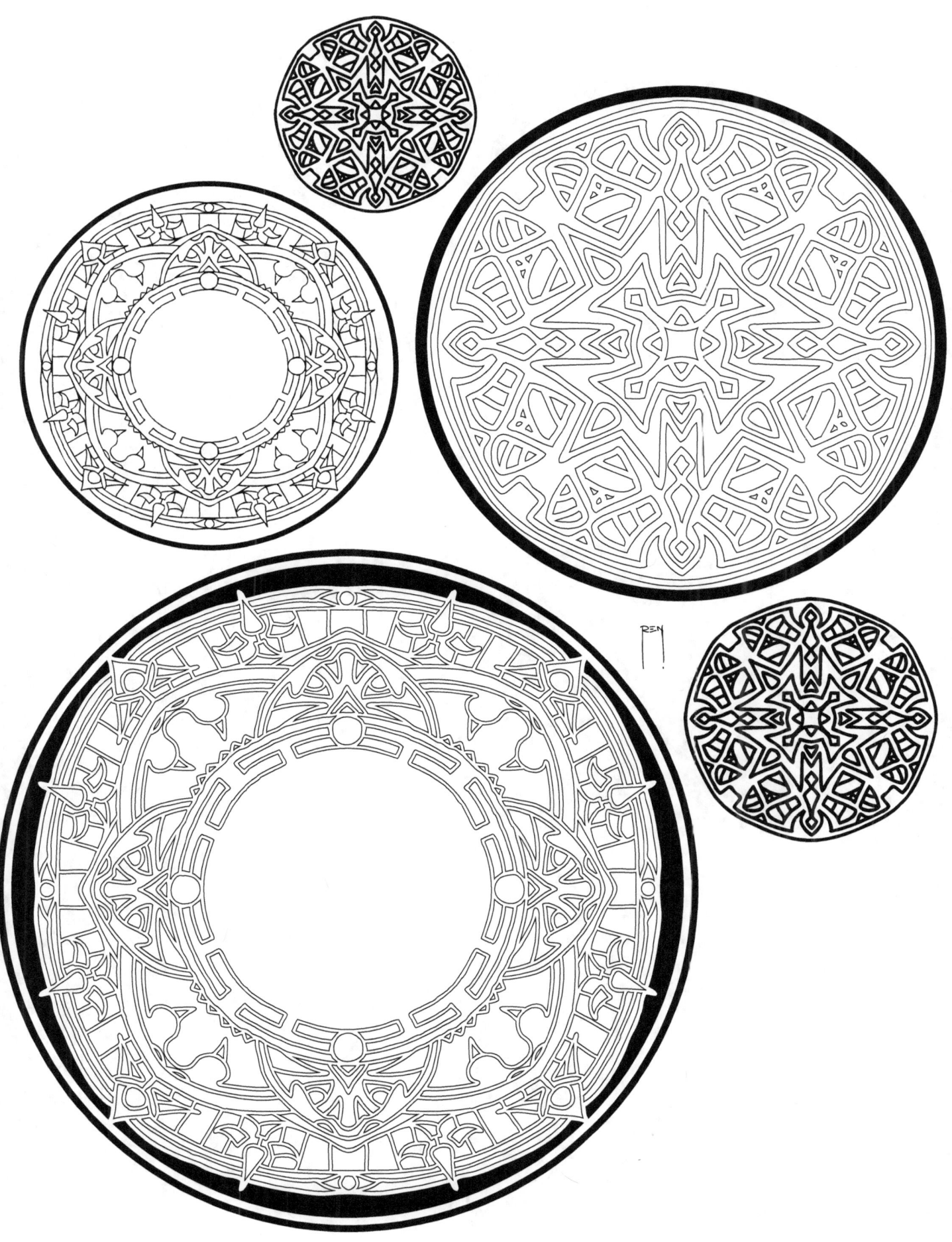

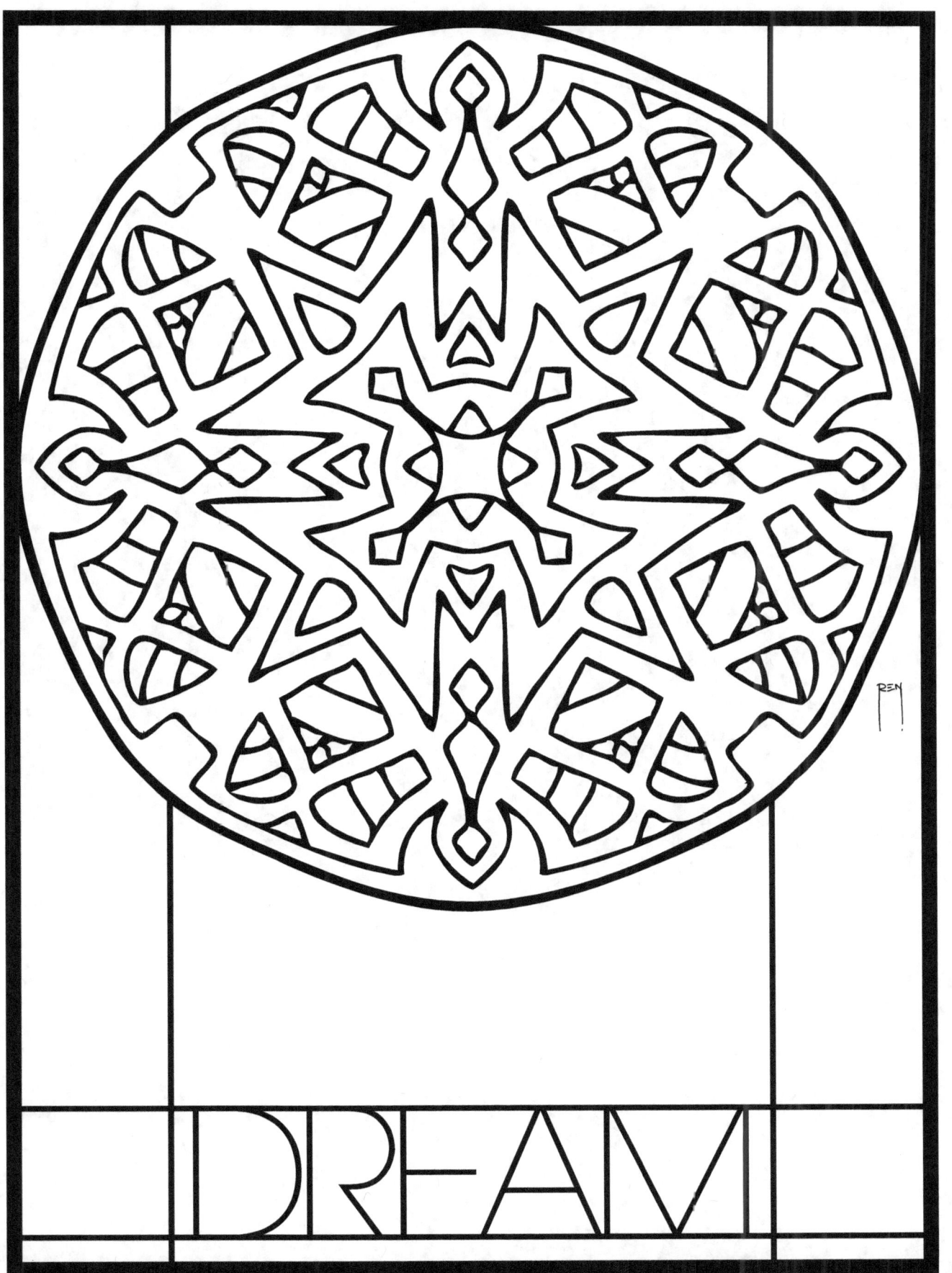

DREAM

Idea: Gaze upon your finished mandala as a form of quiet meditation; this is especially relaxing just before bedtime

Keep a dream journal: before you sleep, write a list of things you'd like to dream about; when you wake, write a list of what you actually dreamt.

Fires that Purify

Walking on Coals Beneath Burning Bridges

As a child in Hawai`i, I was introduced to lava — and Pele, goddess of fire — at a young age. We were taught her power by seeing how she swallowed the sticks and pebbles we threw into the gently flowing puddle of red and black liquid. Later, as a teenager, my apartment in Atlanta caught fire, and my roommates and I had to evacuate. Then, as an adult, my country home in rural Georgia was burnt to blackness. Even away from the islands, Pele reminds me that I am one of her children. Though each fire brought loss, they also propelled me forward and onward in life. Pele teaches us in ways that seem tragic at first, but ultimately, her crucible burns away our weaknesses, our illusions, and our artificial bonds to material things. Her fires make us resilient, mindful, and pure.

Every one of us goes through a crucible; we must all overcome obstacles in life in order to become better, stronger people.

What were some of the fires, whether metaphorical or literal, that occurred in your life? What were some of the impurities that were burnt away, and in what ways did your fires change you? If you feel that you have had to endure more fires than the people around you, write about it on a piece of paper. And then, very carefully, burn it.

Idea:
Print or transfer mandalas onto fabric, and then appliqué onto yoga bags, tote bags, or reusable shopping bags

If you are young, spend an afternoon with an older person. If you're older, then spend the afternoon with a young person. Learn something new from a different generation.

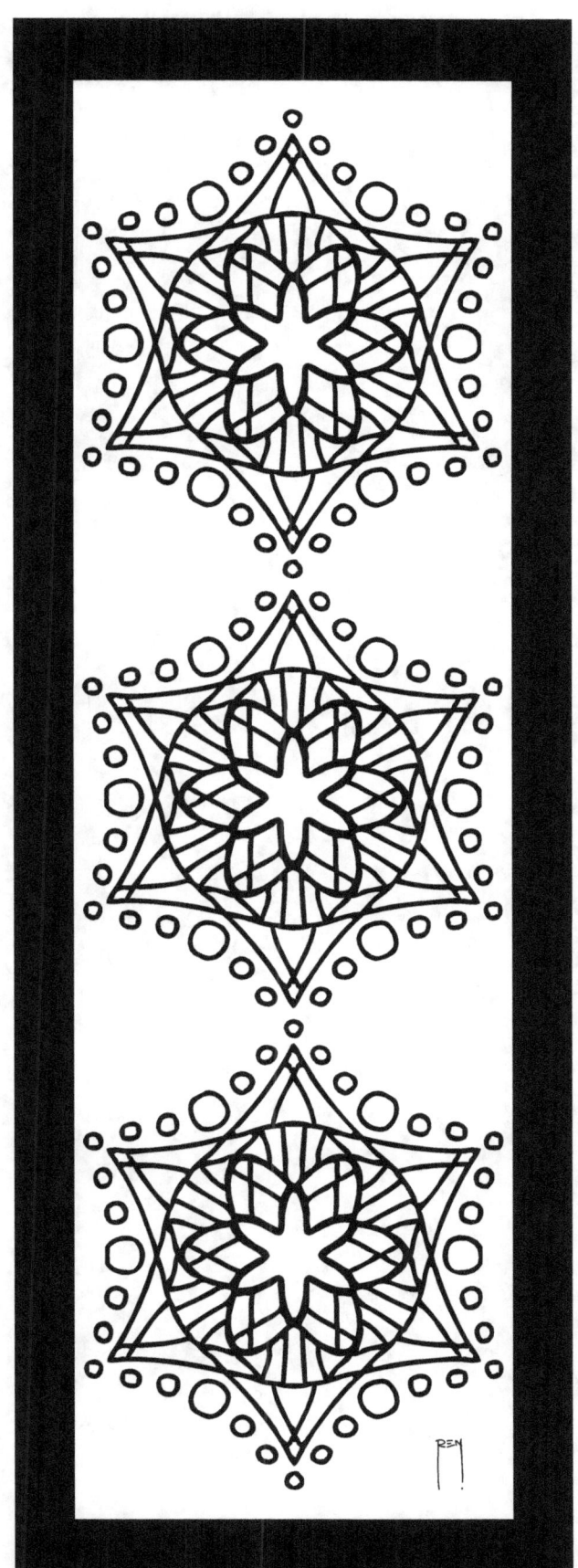

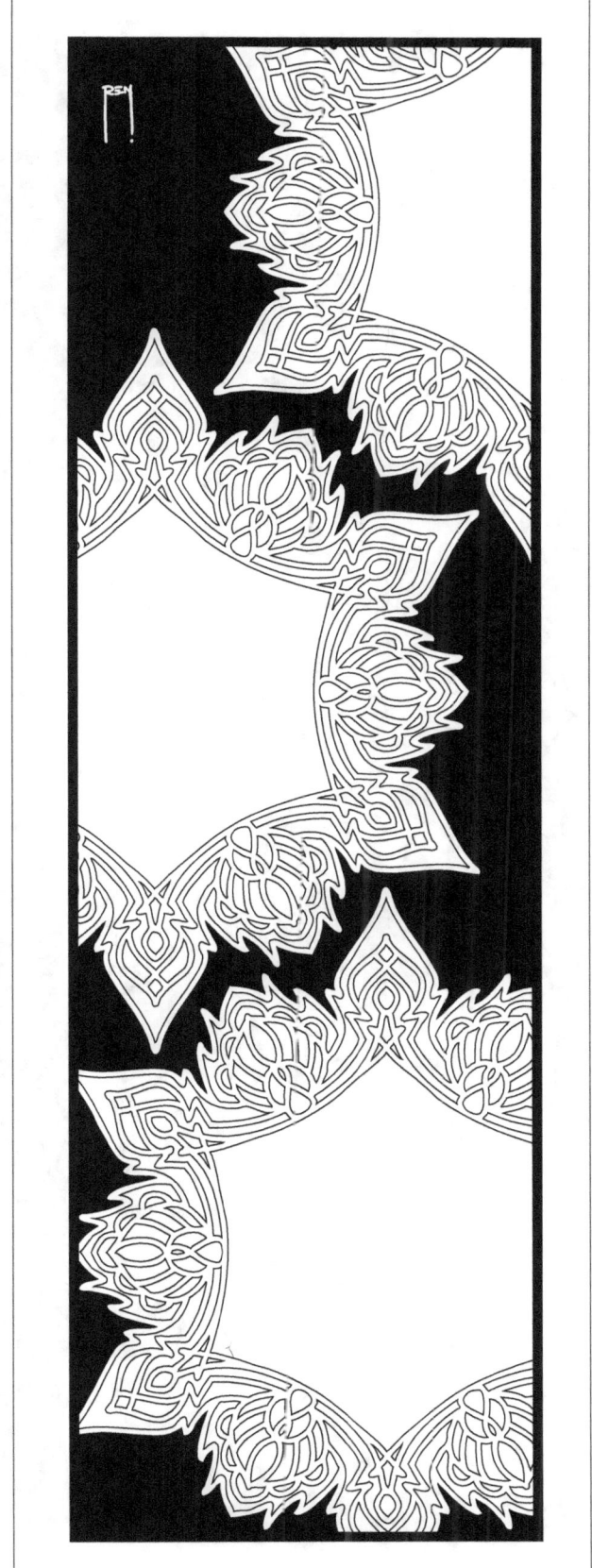

Your imagination is one of life's greatest gifts. Use it.

Idea: Display finished bookmarks as miniature paintings in unexpected places; for example, tape to the side of your computer monitor or on the inside of a cabinet door

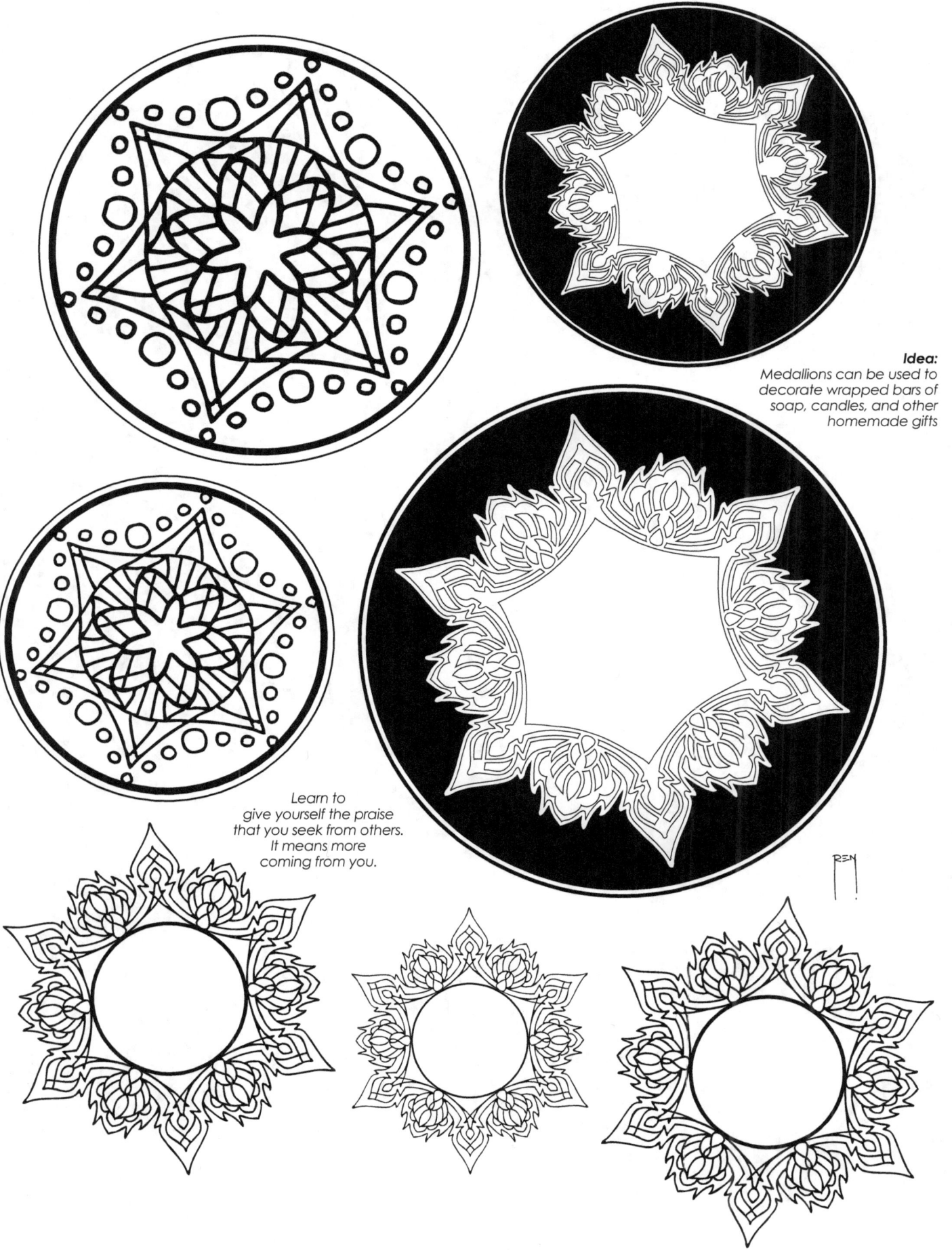

Idea:
Medallions can be used to decorate wrapped bars of soap, candles, and other homemade gifts

Learn to give yourself the praise that you seek from others. It means more coming from you.

CHILDREN OF THE ELEMENTS

A Universal Alchemy

In traditional Chinese medicine, it is believed that our bodies possess qualities of five elements: wood; fire; earth; metal; and water. Basically, if these elements are off balance, then they must be harmonised; or, if they are balanced, then you're golden, so to speak.

In Europe's Middle Ages, alchemists believed that all matter on earth is composed of different combinations of fire, earth, air, and water; and that matter can be "transmuted," or become something completely different (e.g. gold or healing elixirs), by altering its elemental composition. Meanwhile, in India, Ayurvedic health practises include the same four elements, plus the addition of ether, the most subtle and mystical of the five elements.

In these, and many other cultures, the concepts of harmony, growth, and life are the results of balancing the elements; while disharmory, illness, and death are the results of imbalance. We even use elements to describe people: someone can be fiery; earthy; an airhead; a tall (or long) drink of water; etc.

To what elements do you relate the most, and why?

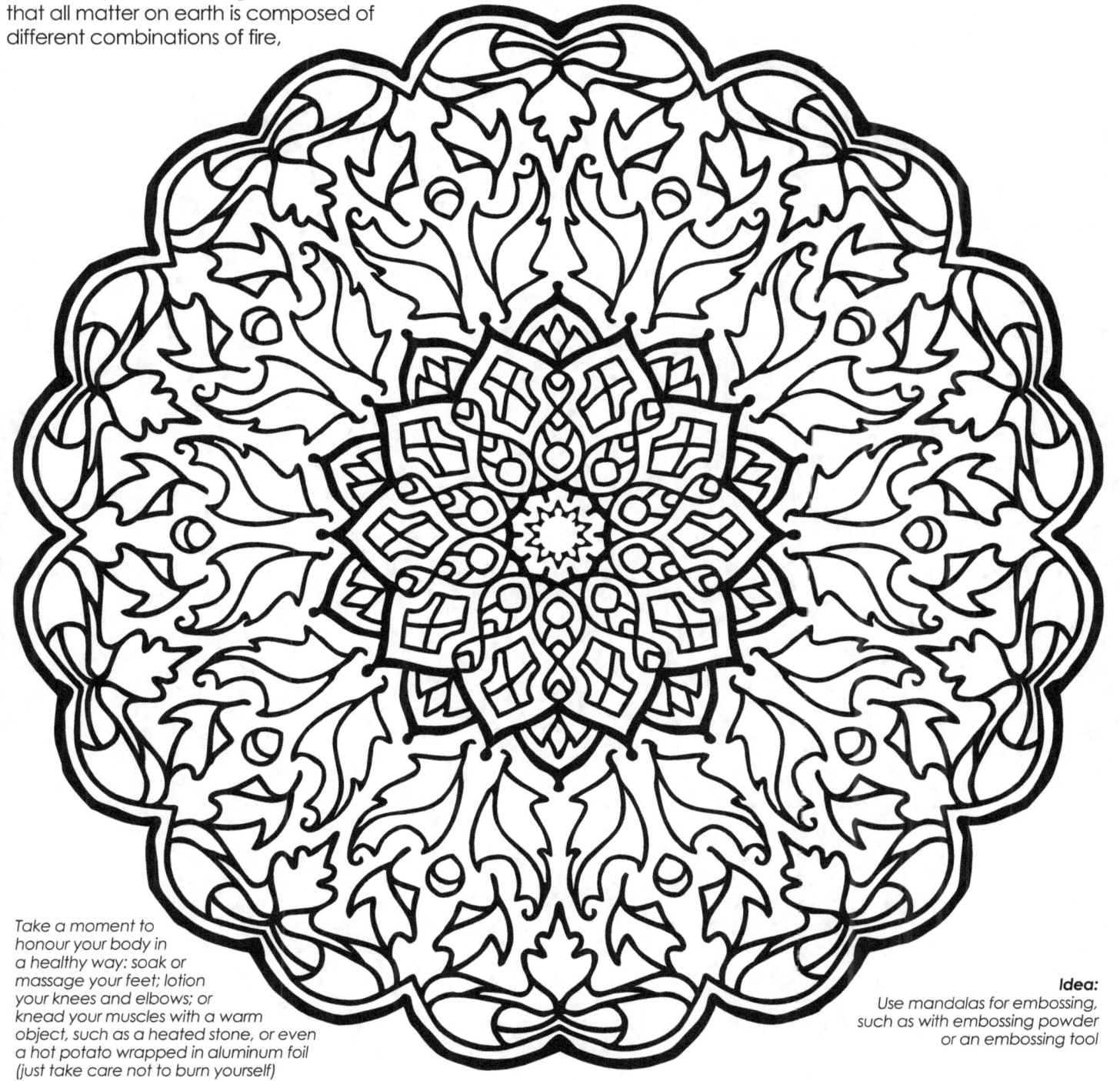

Take a moment to honour your body in a healthy way: soak or massage your feet; lotion your knees and elbows; or knead your muscles with a warm object, such as a heated stone, or even a hot potato wrapped in aluminum foil (just take care not to burn yourself)

Idea:
Use mandalas for embossing, such as with embossing powder or an embossing tool

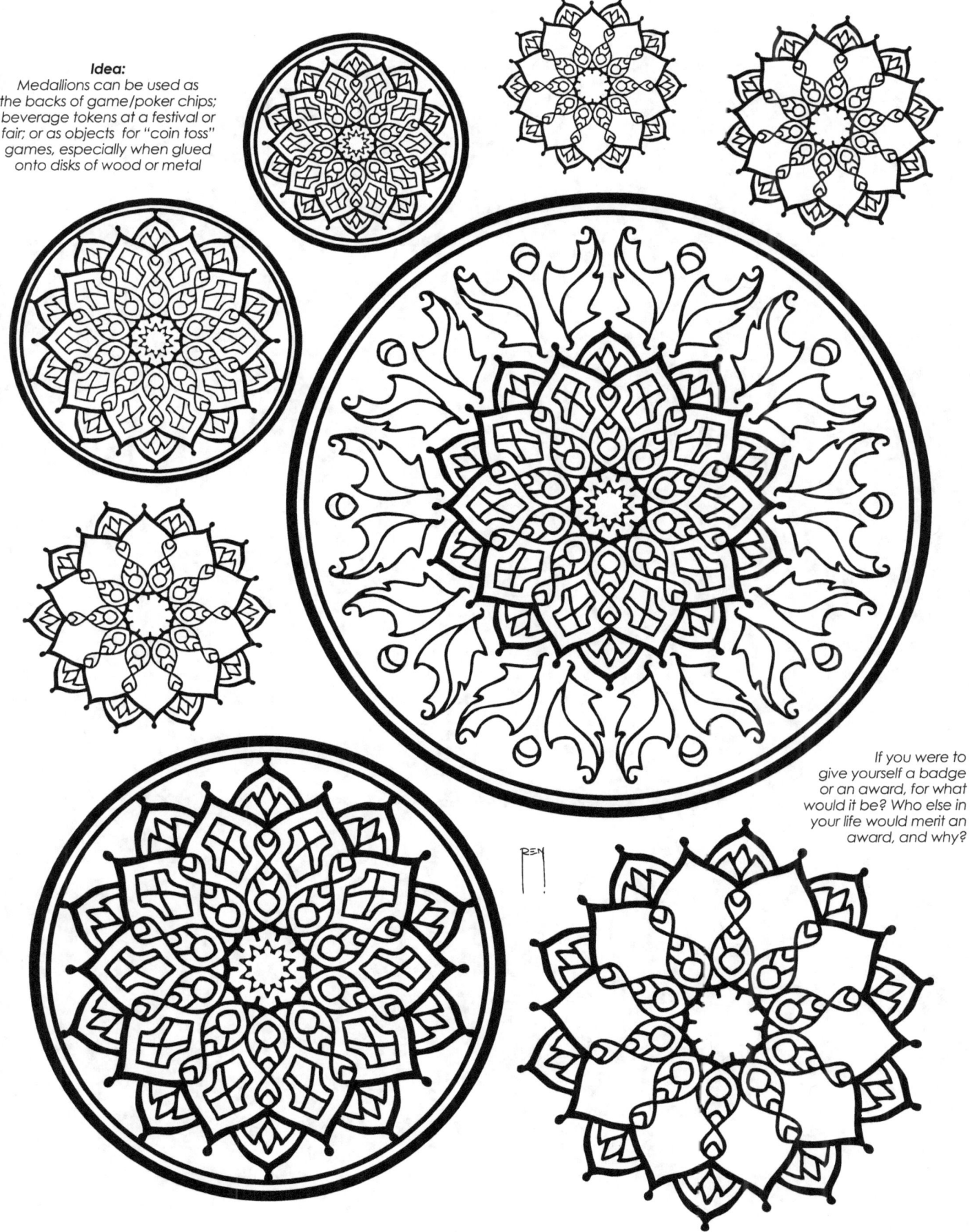

Idea:
Medallions can be used as the backs of game/poker chips; beverage tokens at a festival or fair; or as objects for "coin toss" games, especially when glued onto disks of wood or metal

If you were to give yourself a badge or an award, for what would it be? Who else in your life would merit an award, and why?

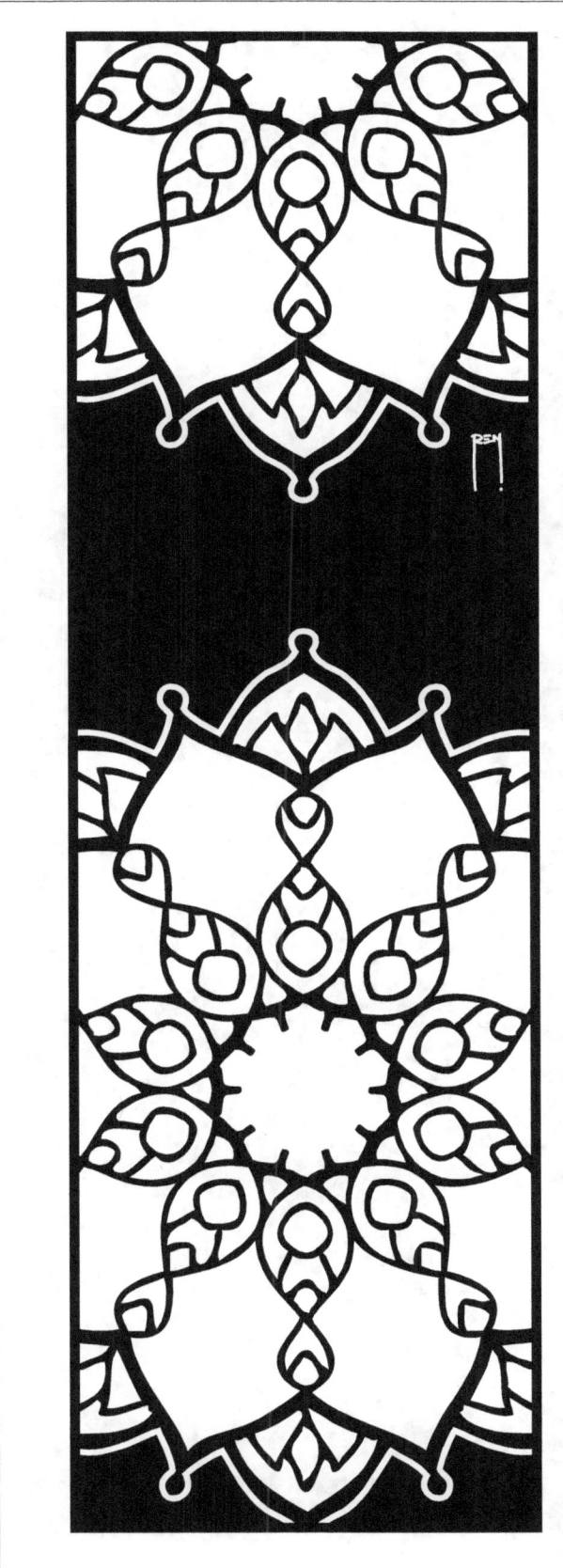

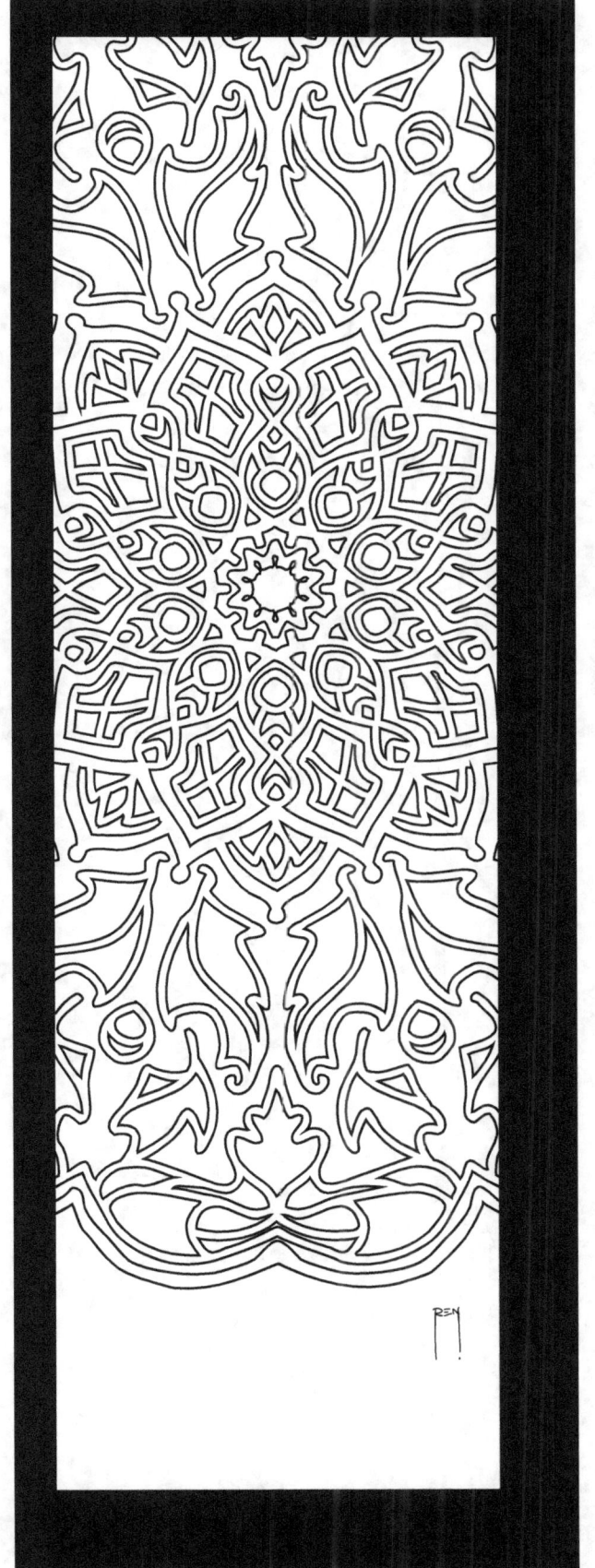

idea: These bookmarks can also be used to decorate the spines of old books

MANIFESTATIONS OF ARMOUR

Different Suits for Different Occasions

21 December 2012 was supposed to be the apocalypse, according to the ancient Mayan calendar, and in the weeks leading up to doomsday, I allowed bloggers, news reporters, and sales figures of candles, bread and milk, and family-sized emergency shelters to let my mind play the "what if?" game, and my "what ifs" were frightening. One of my personal mantras in life is: if something scares you, run towards it. And so I did what any self-respecting, Mayan apocalypse-fearing individual would do while repeating that mantra: I sailed into the Bermuda Triangle. I figured if this was really it, then I may as well have a front-row seat to the event like a V.I.P.

The Triangle was especially stormy that year; even the local islanders commented on the unusually cold and stormy weather. And besides the nightly odd lights over the ocean towards the heart of the Triangle, it was — thankfully — an uneventful doomsday.

To combat fear, one of my types of armour manifests itself in the form of humour. I'd rather be laughing than screaming, and so I find or create opportunities to laugh.

How about you: what kind of armour do you wear when you're afraid? Or sad? Or hurt? Or in love? Or too polite when you don't have to be? How many kinds of armour do you have?

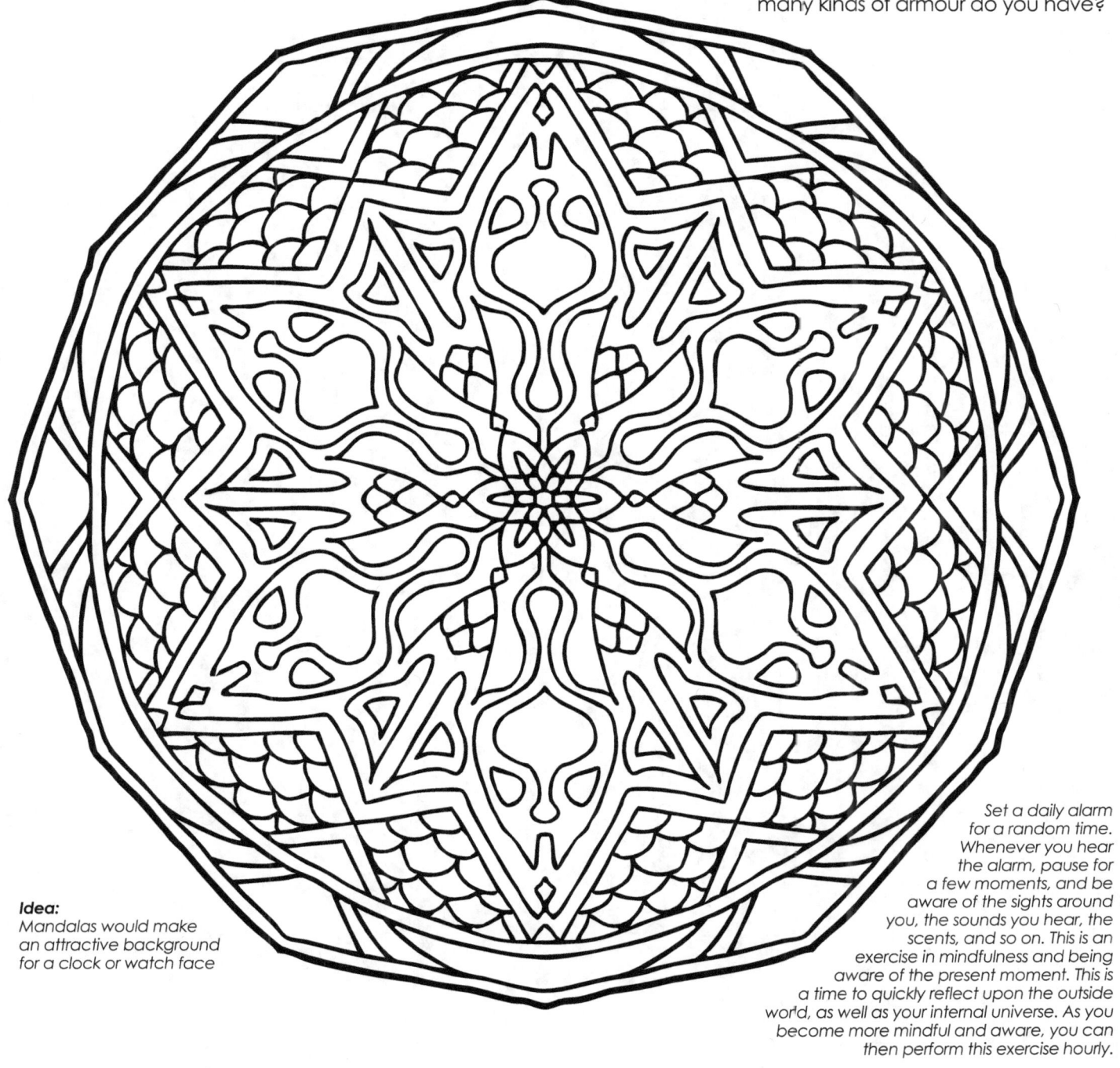

Idea:
Mandalas would make an attractive background for a clock or watch face

Set a daily alarm for a random time. Whenever you hear the alarm, pause for a few moments, and be aware of the sights around you, the sounds you hear, the scents, and so on. This is an exercise in mindfulness and being aware of the present moment. This is a time to quickly reflect upon the outside world, as well as your internal universe. As you become more mindful and aware, you can then perform this exercise hourly.

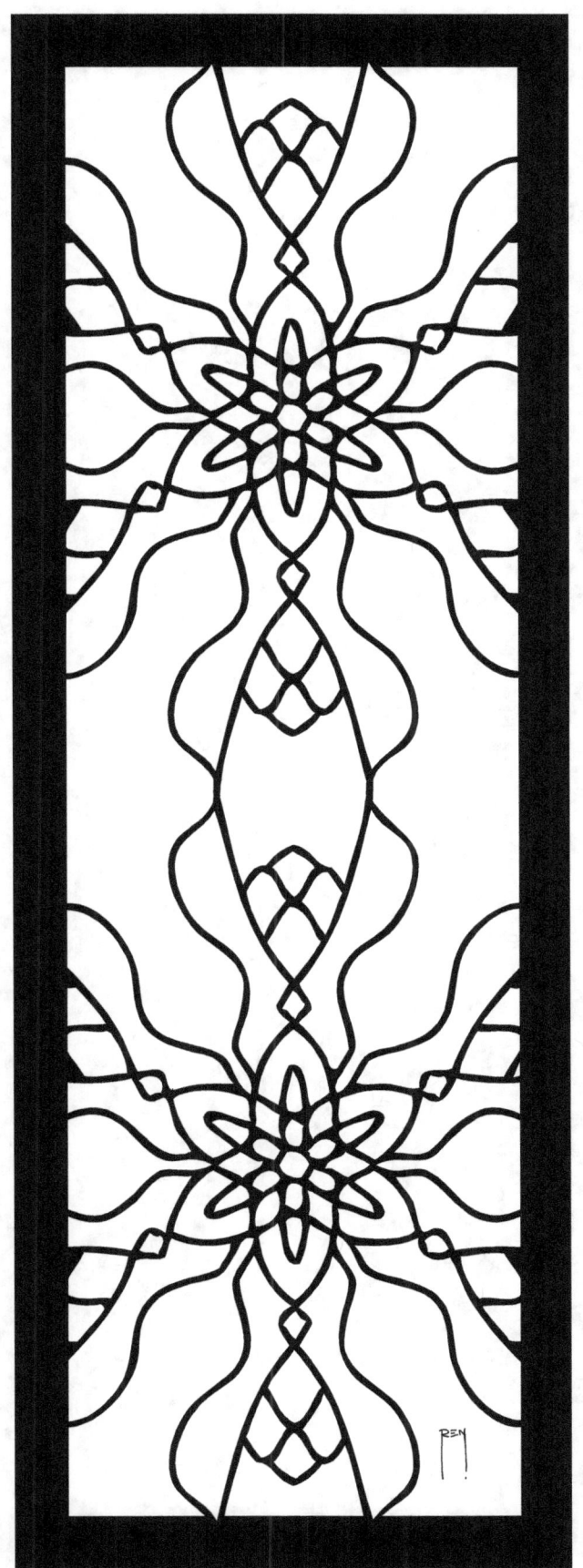

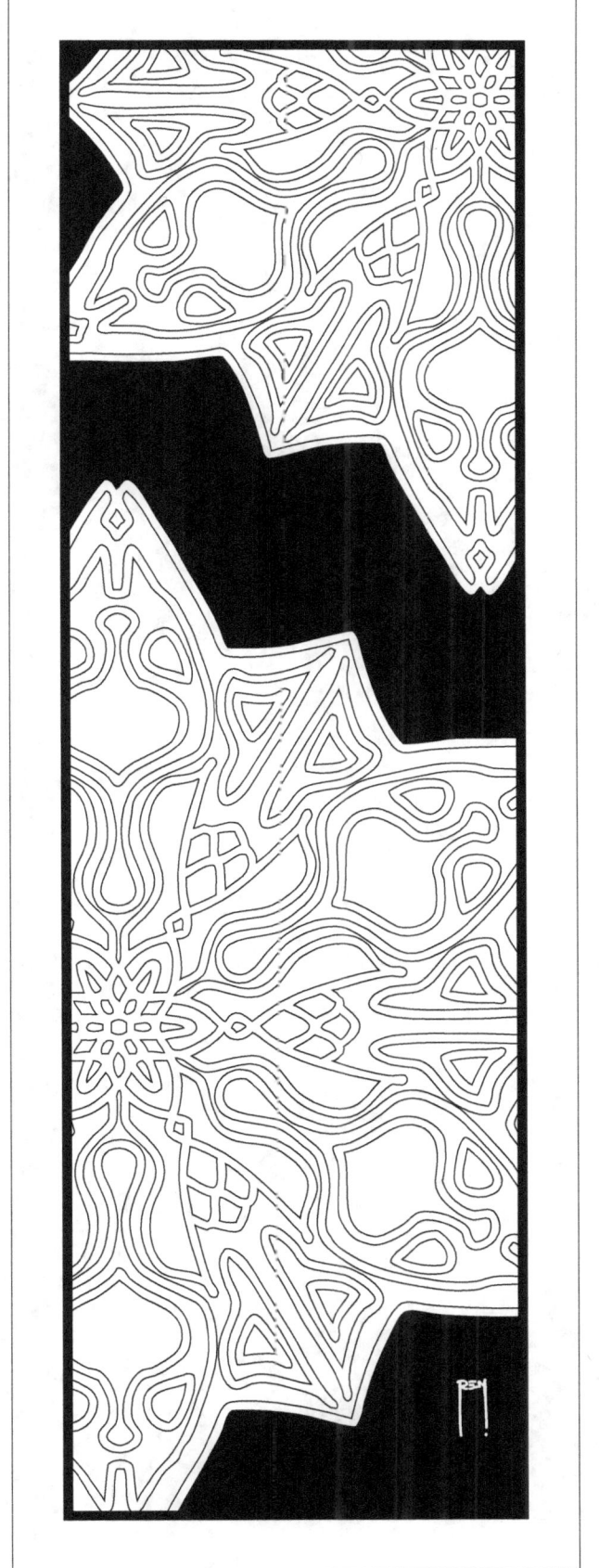

A friend is someone who can get past your armour and reach your heart.

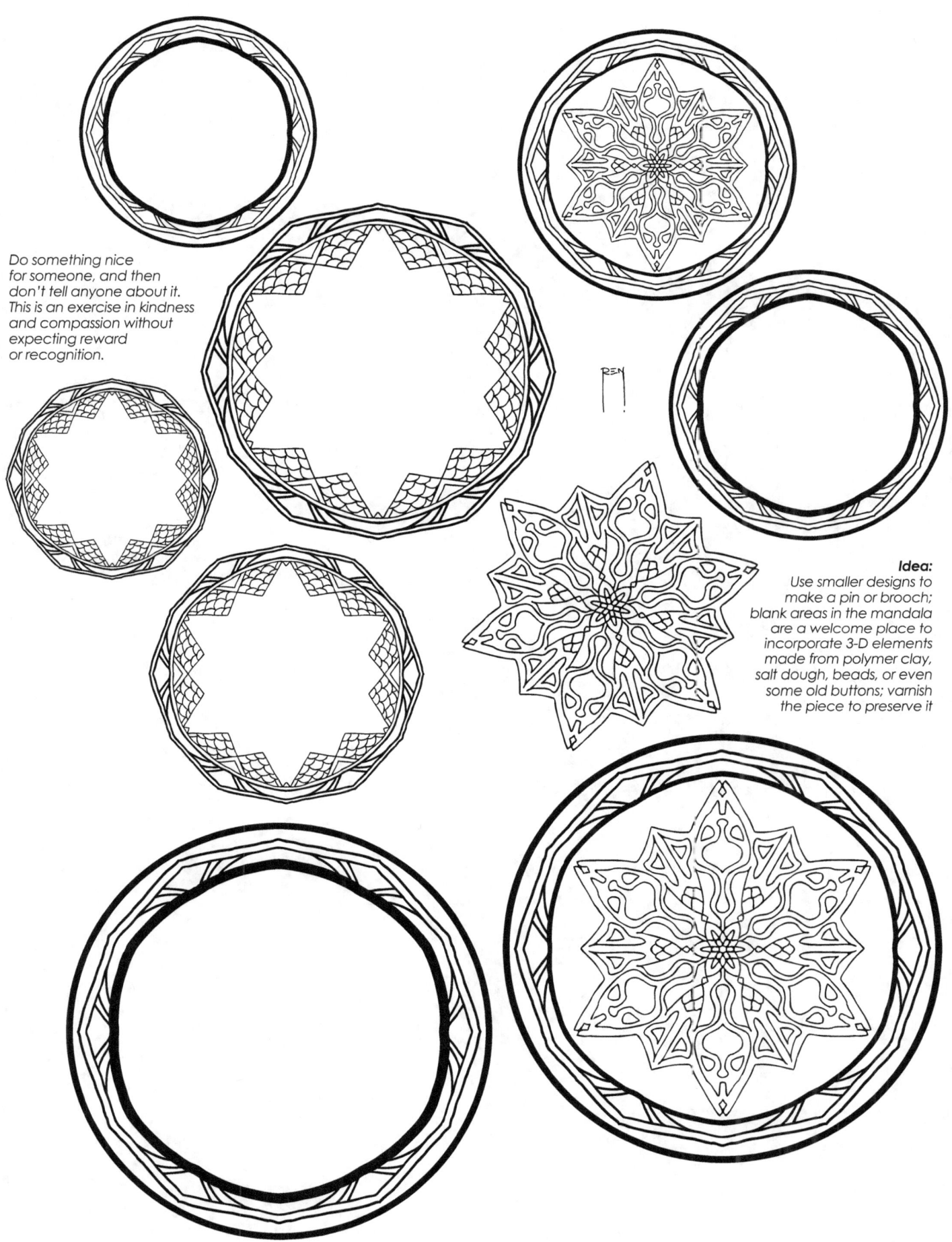

Do something nice for someone, and then don't tell anyone about it. This is an exercise in kindness and compassion without expecting reward or recognition.

Idea:
Use smaller designs to make a pin or brooch; blank areas in the mandala are a welcome place to incorporate 3-D elements made from polymer clay, salt dough, beads, or even some old buttons; varnish the piece to preserve it

Idea:
If you reuse cylindrical containers, like the ones used for oatmeal or some old fashioned candies, then glue or tape a mandala onto the round plastic lid for an attractive cover

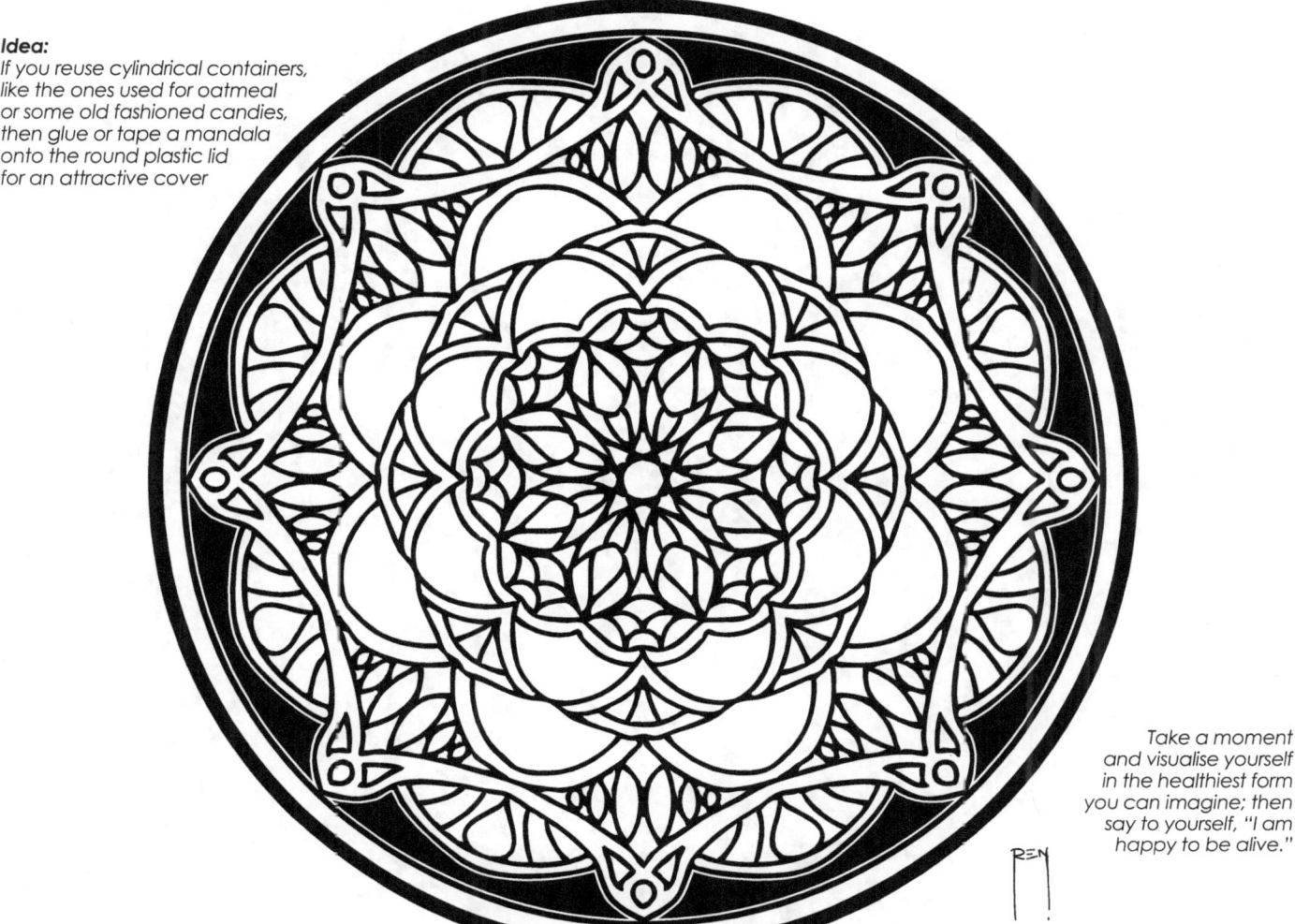

Take a moment and visualise yourself in the healthiest form you can imagine; then say to yourself, "I am happy to be alive."

ABOUT THE AUTHOR & ARTIST

General information

Ren is a writer and visual artist currently based in Southern California. He works in a variety of media in illustration, painting, and sculpture. Outside of fine art, Ren is an award winning graphic designer and advertising art and creative director. He is also a public speaker on subjects ranging from creativity, creative inspiration and instruction, motivational topics, and his experience with TBI (traumatic brain injury) and memory loss.

Ren studied literature and fine arts in France and America; he holds a Bachelor of Fine Arts degree with a focus on the psychology of colour & design.

Artistic influences

Ren's main influences come from his diverse cultural and ethnic heritage: he is Pacific Islander, Asian, and Mediterranean; and his ancestors were Catholic, Buddhist, animist, shamanist, Muslim, Hindu, and Sephardic Jewish. These sensibilities and religious and spiritual symbolism find their way into Ren's art on both a conscious and unconscious level. Language is another influence in his work, as his first language was Hawaiian Creole English; and his most prominent literary influences are the ancient love poetry of India, China, Japan, Egypt, and Sumer. Many of his visual art pieces incorporate the written word and/or typographic design, such as the *Master Mandalas* series of books.

A creative & a servant

The word "Ren" is a Confucian virtue that signifies altruism, or love for others. The writer/artist Ren has chosen this as his professional name as a symbolic way to dissolve the ego and selfish intent during the creative process; therefore, every piece of Ren's art comes from a place of generosity towards, and reverence for, others.

Though Ren is descended from the royal families of the ancient lakanate of Tondo and the sultanates of Sulu and Brunei, he embraces the idea that anyone who acts with kindness and selflessness, listens with respect and open heart, and speaks with thought and honesty is a true royal, regardless of one's upbringing. He believes the best way to honour his ancestors is to help empower others through his art and writing, and to be of service to those in need of compassion and healing. In this way, he strives to contribute to the artistic enrichment of the cultures of the Philippines, Hawai`i, France, and the American Deep South — all places he calls home.

Ren has actively and continuously volunteered his time, effort, fine art, and commercial art work to numerous charitable and humanitarian causes since the age of eight. Learn more about the artist and his work at **RenCollection.org**.

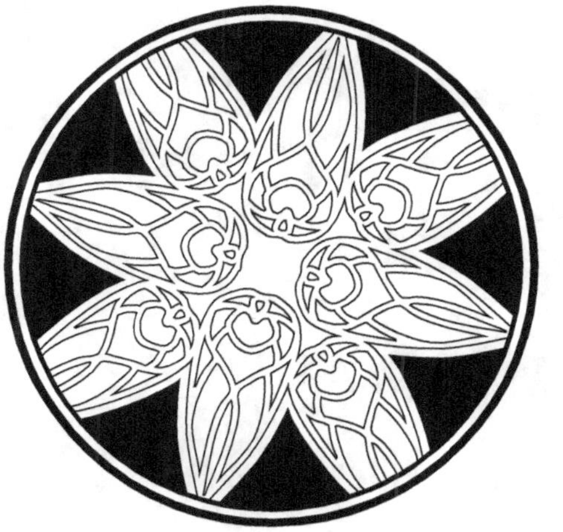

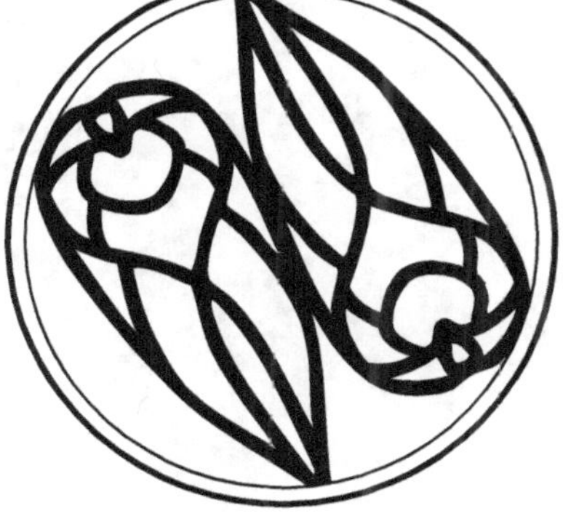

Mahalo, Merci, Salamat, & Thanks, Y'all

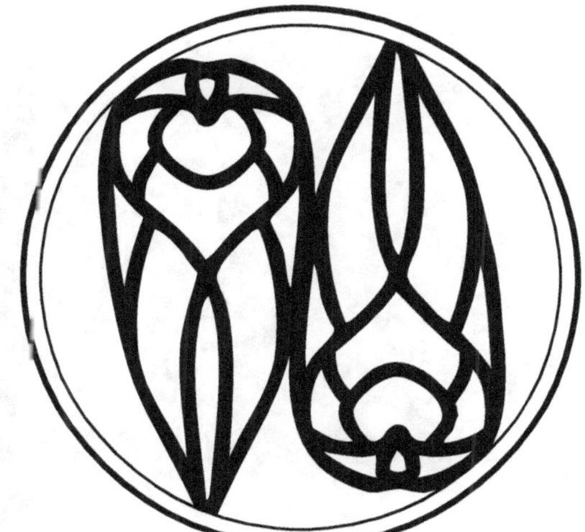

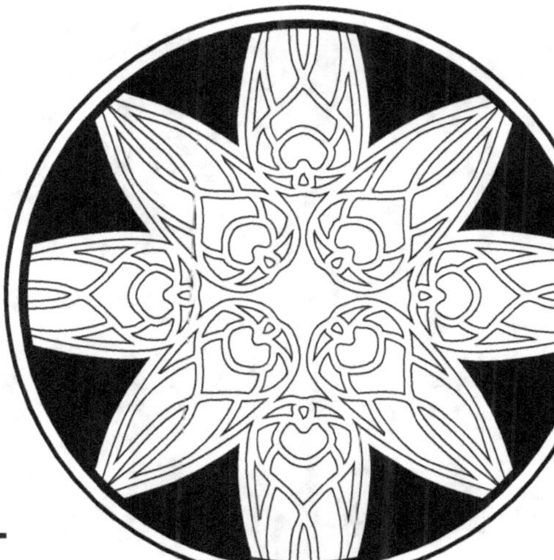

For Supporting Artistic Expression

Thank you for purchasing this edition of *Master Mandalas!*
If you enjoyed this book, the best way to keep it alive is by telling your friends,
family, caregivers, patients, educators, students, and more about *Master Mandalas.*
By spreading the word, you'll be bringing a little colour into their lives
and maybe even helping some of them to heal as well.

*Please note that we are a small organisation, and any unauthorised copying
and distribution of this book and its contents truly does hurt us. We thank you for
honouring our copyright by using this content for personal, non-commercial use only.*

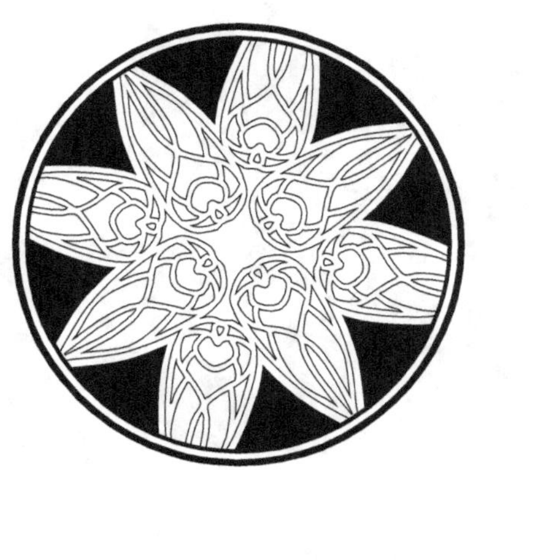

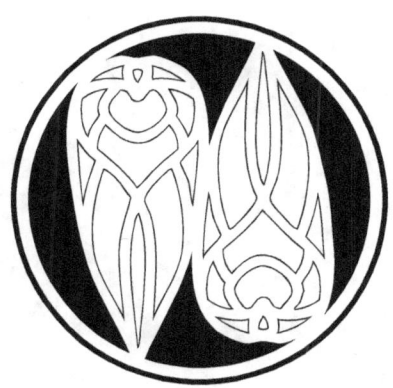  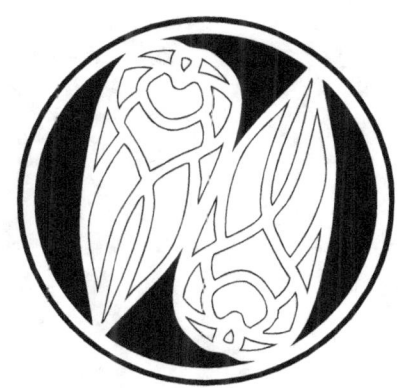